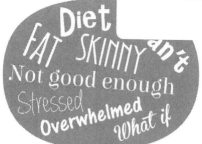

think straight lose weight

the revolutionary way to regain control
and create the body you love

DAVID X GODFREY

RƎTHINK PRESS

First published in Great Britain 2017
by Rethink Press (www.rethinkpress.com)

© Copyright David X Godfrey

CONTENTS

Foreword

Some experts say that weight loss should be easy. We all get taught to just eat less and move more. If this were really the case, why are we in an obesity epidemic and have more disordered eating than ever before?

For as long as I can remember – since school, throughout university, my career as a physiotherapist, to where I am today running two health and fitness companies – I hear stories of women who are lost, confused and frustrated. Completely let down by the diet and fitness industry and left in a place of despair, desperation and a pit of low self-esteem. Food is a source of both pain and comfort.

Having worked with thousands of women over the years, there are common and distinct behavioural patterns that explain *why* women struggle to succeed in long term fat loss or body transformations, none of which have anything to do with food or dieting.

Social media and modern technology have bred a population addicted to instant gratification, conditioned to compare themselves to others, and desiring extravagance. We also have the evolution of the successful, driven woman who not only thinks they can do it all, but feels pressured to be all things to all people.

Today, women struggle with perfectionism and overwhelm; they hugely over-analyse their every move. They worry about what other people think of them, worry about doing things wrong, constantly compare themselves to their favourite Instagram idols and struggle with people pleasing. They are unhappy.

In each of these categories the prevalence of women who secretly struggle with food, control and the feeling of not being good enough - is *out of control!* We have a weight loss problem that is far greater than just solving it with 'Eat Less, Move More'.

This book is for you, my friend: the one who technically has 'all their shit together' on the outside, but on the inside you have hidden secrets. You punish yourself or reward yourself with food. Food controls you: you start a new diet on Mondays, you see foods as good or bad, you fall off the wagon and get back on. Maybe you are now just frustrated and stuck. You have tried a thousand diets and consulted countless 'experts' yet you still cannot lose weight.

Welcome to *Think Straight Lose Weight!*

For long term weight loss, we must look at the bigger picture. The women who are successful long term in weight loss do not just learn about calories, they learn about themselves. Weight loss begins when you are able to manage your emotions, be kinder and have more respect for yourself. You are worth it, you just forgot because of all the nasty things you say to yourself.

Easy to say but how do you actually *do* that?

If it were as easy as shoehorning another diet or exercise program into your already chaotic life, you probably wouldn't be reading this book.

Lifelong weight loss necessitates looking inward, and at the rest of your life first. Unfortunately, this is hard and it cannot be measured using rules or calories, which is why most women don't go there!

You are reading this because you know you deserve more and you are now prepared to do the hard yards for it.

One of my dominant values as a coach has been to

serve at the highest level. I seek out other coaches, doctors and practitioners that I can partner with to make profound and lasting changes. At the top of that list of partners is David.

David's ability to create long term life changes in his clients is nothing short of amazing. His unique, professional and nurturing approach to the most serious of cases frequently leaves me thinking, 'How the hell do you do that? How do you know what to do and say to illicit that degree of behavioural change?'

I am lucky enough to have him as my business partner in Chase Life and as a team we have transformed lives and created long term fat loss results that I dreamed about when I started my career. Above all, as my husband I also see the other side. The dedication, work and commitment that he gives every client, the behind-the-scenes conversations we have to ensure the best in business practice, client care and service.

Finally, with this book *Think Straight Lose Weight*, you will be able to uncover the secrets of how David works, start implementing new methods into your life to lose weight, become happier and wave goodbye to stress, perfectionism, anxiety and worry.

Ladies, we have lost our way and it's time to take back control! Embrace change, learn vulnerability and know we have complete ownership of our destiny. It's time to *Think Straight* and *Lose Weight*.

Rachel Guy
Director, Athletic Fox Ltd
Director, Chase Life Ltd

Introduction

When somebody wants a physical transformation they typically focus all their energy and attention on diet and exercise. Whilst these are important, they are just the tip of the iceberg. It has been said that business success is 80% mindset and 20% strategy. Similar quotes have been referenced in sport, and it applies to fat loss and body transformations too. Diet and exercise matter, but they are supported by your mindset, the way you organise your thoughts and your life.

Most people fail in their body transformation attempts because they struggle to follow their diet, lose motivation, lose self-belief, or create so much stress through overwhelm, low self-esteem, perfectionism, or anxiety that their body and mind end up working against them.

Unfortunately, the typical response is to spend yet more time and energy searching for another diet or training programme, the one that will sort everything out. But there isn't one. These issues are purely mindset based, and that is where the solutions lie.

Even if you have struggled for years with your weight, body image, or with compulsive behaviours and self-sabotage, you can turn this around in a very short space of time. You can create a lean, fit, healthy, body, *and* be happy, confident, and fulfilled at the same time. I have dedicated my career to delivering this for my clients.

Many people believe that overcoming some of the issues I have mentioned, and making personal changes of this nature, is a long and painful process. Nothing could be further from the truth. You don't have to drag up problems from the past. You don't have to beat yourself up. You don't have to suffer for years. Personal change can happen in an instant, and as you will discover, it can and should be great fun! The strategies of success in any endeavour tap into your true sense of purpose, bring out the best in you, amplify your motivation, give you supreme confidence, and make you feel excited and passionate about yourself, your life, and your journey. Sure, there is a lot of work to be done, but it is exhilarating work, it's what makes you feel alive and that you are winning at the game of life.

Everything I talk about in this book is vital to your body transformation success. Some of the topics will be obvious: motivation, or resolving binge eating. Others – such as setting goals for a happy and fulfilling life in other areas including your career, relationships, and life purpose – are less so. These are all interconnected. The more integrated and aligned your thoughts, emotions, and life as a whole, the more successful you will become in every aspect - including your body transformation. Unhappy, stressed people who lack balance or purpose, or who suffer with internal conflicts, are unlikely to make any kind of sustainable body transformation.

Once you make the internal changes I will guide you through in this book you will discover that building a fit, lean, healthy body becomes very simple; a normal, natural, integral part of who you are and what you do every day. It becomes a part of you, something that is aligned with your beliefs, your values, your core sense of identity, as well as your life as a whole.

However, personal change of this nature does not just happen, and does not come purely from an intellectual understanding. It is a neurological event, something you have to feel in your body and your nervous system. I could describe in intimate detail what it's like to go skydiving, but you will only know what I am talking about when you jump out of the plane. Reading this book is not enough. Understanding why you have struggled in the past and what you need to do differently to transform your future is not enough. You must do the work. You must apply yourself to every one of the exercises and techniques I will guide you through, and commit to them fully until you create the internal changes I describe.

You cannot get the changes you want through a treatment, pill, or surgery. If you want to get fit, you must train. If you want to stay fit, you must continue to train. Your mind is similar. We are conditioning ourselves every day. Put in the work now, and maintaining that condition in the future becomes easy – just a natural, habitual part of your routine. This is how you will create the body you want, and love your life at the same time.

Know What You Want

What You Will Learn

» The structure of motivation.

» Why traditional goal-setting has failed to help you transform your body.

» Why people can't stick to a diet or exercise programme.

» The core reasons why people yo-yo or seem to lack consistency.

» How to get yourself motivated and truly excited about your goals.

» How to programme your unconscious to prevent self-sabotage, and keep you motivated and on track *when it matters most.*

» How to design a life that supports and enhances your body goals.

» How to ensure that all your goals are aligned and work synergistically together instead of against one another.

What Don't You Want?

Too many people fail to get what they want in life because they don't know what they want. Especially in their fitness, health and body goals.

Everyone knows what they *don't* want. They don't want their gut hanging over their belt. They don't want to feel self-conscious. They don't want to feel like food controls them anymore.

They may also have things they are afraid of happening in the future. Perhaps they are afraid their children will follow their example and lead unhealthy lives. Or that if they don't lose weight their health, relationships or another area of their life will suffer.

Many fitness journeys are initiated by these types of emotions. We call this **Push motivation**. You are motivated to eliminate or avoid something, either now or in the future.

Push motivation is useful and powerful as it initiates action. Indeed, the majority of people are more motivated by pain in the beginning than by pleasure. For example, would you be more motivated to earn £100k, or to prevent someone from stealing £100k from you? Most people are more motivated by the latter.

Whilst Push motivation is excellent for creating action, many people embark on a journey to improve their life (whether it's their body, or finances, or something else) with Push motivation the only motivation they are clear about. Unfortunately, as you progress away from your pain, your Push motivation correspondingly reduces. All of a sudden it doesn't seem so important to attend that gym session or to prepare your healthy meals for the next day.

What Do You Want?

At the other end of the spectrum it is critical that you know precisely *what* you do want and *why* you want it. This is called **Pull motivation**. Pull motivation is what you are attracted to have, feel, experience or do more of in your life. In contrast to Push motivation, Pull motivation increases the more progress you make towards it. As you start to notice progress, and experience better and better results each week, the positive reinforcement increases your excitement and motivation. You begin seeing, hearing, and feeling the benefits of all your hard work.

Unfortunately, most people have impotent goals. They have vague ideas like "I want to lose weight", or "I'd like to be in better shape" or my personal favourite, "I just want to tone up a bit"!

For a goal to be motivating you need to be able to picture it vividly, describe it in precise detail, and experience it in your mind as if it were real. Crucially, the internal experience you have when you imagine it needs to be truly exciting for you.

First of all, for a goal to be motivating it needs to fit the SMART acronym. I know, you've heard it all a million times already! The SMART acronym is still relevant, but is often misunderstood and incomplete, which is why many people fail to make it work properly.

For a goal to be effective and motivating it needs to be SMART:

S pecific

M easureable

A chievable

R ealistic

T ime-framed

SMART Mistakes

Specific and Measurable

"I want to lose weight" is too vague. "I want to be 15% body fat" or "I want to be 130lbs" is both specific and measurable. But unfortunately, it is not specific enough for what you really want. What is your ultimate goal as a result of achieving 15% body fat or 130lbs? Most people want to look and feel good.

Two people with the same body fat percentage can look very different. But even the same person can look vastly different at the same body fat percentage, since physical appearance also depends on muscle size and shape, the proportions of muscles relative to each other, posture, and general health and wellbeing.

Tape and body fat measurements are nevertheless useful indicators of the direction you are heading in, and you will generally see changes in these numbers faster than in your physical appearance. By all means, use them as an overall guide, but recognise that they are still a step removed from what you *really* want.

Photographs are a much more accurate representation of what you want to measure: changes in your appearance. But how can you ensure your goals are Specific and Measurable if photographs are your primary method for measuring progress? You need to get clearer and describe what you want to create. Do you want to see the indentation to the sides of your abdominals? Do you want to see the line between your deltoids (shoulders) and triceps (upper arm)? Do you want your buttocks to be rounder, higher and firmer?

Achievable, Realistic and Time-Framed

Most people don't know what is achievable. Some people have completely unrealistic expectations. They want to create the body of an athlete – which takes years of consistent and focused training and nutrition - in the space of a few months, after years and years of unhealthy living.

Other people choose goals that are too small. They don't realise they can achieve so much more, because their expectations are based on the fact that, until now, it has felt like such a struggle. This results in unexciting goals (to be discussed below).

Others want what they can't have. Everyone can get lean, but there are some things you can't change. If you have short limbs and are naturally curvy, you are never going to achieve the long, slender figure of a catwalk model. So your goals need to be based on becoming the very best version of you.

To discover what is achievable and realistic in the timeframe you have set for yourself, your best bet is to consult an expert – someone who has experience in creating sustainable transformations. Whilst they won't be able to predict precisely how long it will take you, they will be able to guide you as to whether your expectations are reasonable or not.

Progress Expectations

The biggest mistake people make with regards to realistic expectations relates to their expectations of the *journey*. You *will* plateau, meet obstacles, make mistakes, experience setbacks, and even regress for short periods. You will have to regroup, overcome problems, and find solutions to all the unexpected obstacles you will come across. As the saying goes, find a way, or find an excuse. This is a necessary step on your journey.

SMART TEPER Goals

We also need to add the following to the SMART acronym to make it effective:

Towards language

Towards and Away From language (referred to as positive and negative language in NLP) is a fundamental concept for personal growth and success.

Many people define what they want by what they *don't*

want. This is Away From language. It uses words such as don't, not, less, without, reduce, fewer, etc, to escape something you don't like. Here are some examples:

"I don't want to be *fat*."

"I want to lose *weight*."

"I wish I wasn't so *bothered by what other people think*."

"I want to be less of an *anxious* person."

"I need to reduce my *stress* levels."

"I wish I could lose weight without feeling like *food controls m*e all the time."

Unfortunately, the brain doesn't know how to NOT do something. Try this: don't think of a black cat. Inevitably the first thing your brain thinks of is a black cat. You get more of what you focus on.

In the examples above I have highlighted certain words in *italics*. As you say each of those sentences, your brain identifies what each of those words means and specifically what it means to you. In a later chapter, we will talk about focus and mental rehearsal. Directing your life by what you don't want is like using mental rehearsal to programme your brain to give you more of it!

Instead we need to define our outcomes purely in terms of what we *do* want – what we want to have, feel, experience, and do more of.

Examples of Towards language:

"I want to be lean, fit and healthy."

"I want to feel extraordinary confidence when I talk to new people."

"I want to experience more peace and relaxation throughout the day."

"I want to approach goals and challenges with a strong sense of calm, confidence and self-assurance."

"I want to eat a healthy, nutritious diet that supports my goals, while still enjoying my food, and feeling relaxed around food."

Now your brain knows exactly what you *do* want, and what to focus on in order to give it to you.

Now try changing the word "want" to "will".

Now try changing "I want to be" to "I am", and "I want to feel" to "I feel". More on this later.

For now, remember that to be effective all your goals must be stated in Towards language, and Towards language *only.*

Towards and Away From language doesn't just refer to goal-setting, it affects you from moment to moment.

For example, any time you feel stuck or have a problem ask yourself *"what do I want?"*. You'll notice that your natural tendency is to talk about escaping the problem, what you are worried or afraid of, or what's upsetting you. In other words, you focus on what you don't want, instead of setting clear targets for what you are going to *do* and how you are going to *feel*.

This comes up time and again during our Chase Life programme. Even once someone understands it intellectually, it can take a while to train them out of it. It sounds so simplistic but once you make this switch in how you think it completely transforms your life.

Exciting

As I mentioned above, many people consider for a brief moment what they *really* want, and then tell themselves they can't have it. This is because of fear or limiting beliefs (to be discussed later). Instead they shrink their goals and make them small enough to fit within the limitations they have put upon themselves.

Unfortunately, this results in unexciting, impotent goals that hold little motivational power. When you imagine achieving your diminished goal you think, "Yeah, that would be kind of nice to have". To get you through all those obstacles and challenges we talked about earlier, you need an emotion that is much more powerful than this!

Your goal needs to be truly and genuinely *exciting*. When you imagine your goal, you need to physically feel the excitement in your body and think "Yes! That's what I want, and I can't wait to have it"!

If your goals don't fill you with that level of excitement, you need to go back and design better goals.

Present Tense

When Tom Watson, the founder of IBM, was asked what he attributed the success of IBM to he said:

> *"Firstly, I had a very clear picture of what the company would look like when it was done.*
>
> *Secondly I asked myself how a company which looks like that would have to act.*

And finally, I then realised that unless we began to act that way from the very beginning, we would never get there. In other words, for IBM to become a great company, it would have to act like a great company before it ever became one."

From *The E-Myth* by Michael E Gerber

The same is true of you, your goals, and your life. This is why you should phrase your goals in the present tense, as though you are already that person, living that life, and experiencing those results. Use "I am..." instead of "I will..." or "I want...".

Think, feel, and act today the way that the future you does, and allow time for your body and your physiology to catch up and reflect that image.

Stating your goals in the present tense will also help programme your unconscious mind and your automatic behaviour, which we will discuss in more detail when we come to mental rehearsal.

Emotions

This is the *why* that drives your goals in the first place. What is the *ultimate* reason you want to achieve a goal, whether it be a body transformation, more money, a relationship, or a big house? The answer is because of how you think it will make you feel at the end of it.

Once again these must be stated in Towards rather than Away From language. Many make the mistake of pursuing a physical transformation because they want to escape a negative emotion such as self-conscious-ness, shyness, or insecurity. Using my black cat analogy again, that's like walking around thinking "I hope I'm not thinking of a black cat any more"!

It is vital that in addition to how you want to look and feel *physically*, you identify how you want to feel *emotionally* as a result. It is very sad how frequently we encounter people who achieve the physical transformation they thought was going to make them happy, and they still don't feel any better, because they lost sight of the end goal, *why* they were doing it and what they *really* want. At best, they remain unhappy. At worst, and most frequently, they regress all the way back to their original condition.

Range

Once you have identified a specific physical or financial goal, and how you will measure it, it is a very good idea to have a range within which you allow yourself to fluctuate.

Quite often someone pushes hard to achieve peak condition for an important event such as a wedding, a party, or simply for the summer. After the event, they usually relax to a certain extent, but without setting boundaries on their condition or their behaviour, they will lapse into old habits. Set your peak condition at one end of the range that you will push a bit harder to achieve for those special occasions, and a baseline condition that allows you some flexibility the rest of the time. If at any point you cross that threshold you immediately do what is necessary to get yourself back in range.

The Yo-Yo Effect

So, let's back up a level and return to our discussion on Push and Pull motivation. We have Push motivation, which is the pain we want to avoid, and we have Pull motivation, which is the pleasure we want to add (our SMART TEPER goals). Both are important and have their place, and we will use both to keep you on track.

Once someone is clear on what their Push and Pull motivations are, this still doesn't guarantee they will remain on track to their ultimate goal.

There can come a point when the pain that prompted them to take action in the first place is no longer a daily reminder. Their clothes aren't so tight any more, and they don't feel so self-conscious. However, they aren't close enough to their goal so that they experience daily reminders of what they've achieved, and enjoy the rewards and benefits that come with it.

Their pain doesn't feel so significant, and the pleasure hasn't yet become a big enough daily experience. This is when people start cutting corners. It no longer seems such a big deal to skip a workout, get lazy on food prep, or indulge in off-plan meals.

Before you know it, they are all the way back to Square One again. Now what happens? Their pain ramps up again, they think "how could I have let this happen?" and they get "back on the wagon" again, either with the original plan, or a different diet/workout/fat loss plan, because the other one "didn't work". The cycle repeats itself and they yo-yo back and forth.

This happens in large part because their mindset is reactive and responds to what is happening *in the present moment.* To remain on track, they need to be able to travel back and forth through time in their mind. They need to vividly remember the pain that kick started them in the first place, and vividly imagine their ultimate goal so that it starts to feel real, and truly exciting. Crucially, they need to remind themselves of this pain and pleasure *when it matters most.*

It is important to recognise that the pain and pleasure you feel, the Push and Pull motivation forces in your life, have nothing to do with reality and everything to do with focus.

Push and Pull Competition

It is easy to focus on the Push and Pull motivation related to your physical goal when you are in the gym, when you are reading about nutrition, and when you are talking about diet with your trainer.

But what about when it is the end of a long, stressful day, it's late and the last thing you want to be doing is your meal prep, or going to the gym. Now what are you focusing on? The pain you now associate with working out, and doing your meal prep, and the pleasure you associate with sitting on the couch, with a pizza and a movie. Push and Pull motivators are now guiding you in a completely different direction.

The motivational force that wins is the one you fuel, the one you condition your brain to focus on.

Your long-term success depends on your ability to keep your behaviour consistent, and aligned with your goal. You need to increase the pain and pleasure you associate with achieving your goal to a point that over-whelms any pain and pleasure that could distract you. Then you must link it in your mind to those specific times and situations that, in the past, would have triggered self-sabotage. Let's do this right now.

Exercise: physical Push and Pull motivation

Write down your Push motivation for your physical goal. Write down all the pain you associate with your current condition, as well as what you are afraid of in the future. Make this list detailed and compelling and have the courage to engage with and write down your emotions. The greater the emotions the more powerfully we can programme your mind for success. Remember we need to make this pain greater than any pain that you could potentially associate with not following your goal.

Write down your Pull motivation for your physical goal. This is your SMART TEPER goal. Once again we need to make this pleasure greater than any pleasure that you could associate with not following your goal, so make sure that it is genuinely exciting, focus on emotions, and why this goal is an absolute must for you.

Make a list of the key moments you have gone off track or sabotaged yourself in the past. Identify the most important one, and identify the trigger moment – the first thing you are aware of that used to start the whole sabotage process off. This could be a feeling, something you say to yourself, or a particular situation. In particular, identify *your* involvement in the process – what is the first thing *you* do, say to yourself, imagine, or focus on?

Exercise: Re-patterning

Allocate approximately 10 undisturbed minutes for this exercise.

Close your eyes and imagine the trigger you identified above starting to happen. Do this vividly, but only imagine the beginnings of it.

As soon as you start to get a strong sense of that trigger, immediately transport yourself into the future, to the long-term negative consequences of failing to achieve your goal. Make this experience as unpleasant as possible. How bad would it feel physically? How bad would it feel emotionally? What effect would it have on your pride, your self-esteem, your sense of self? What about other areas of your life: your career, your relationships, your intimate life, your social life? Add details to what you can see, hear, and feel until you feel physical repulsion.

Take on a phenomenally strong, confident posture and facial expression, and in your mind, at the top of your internal voice shout the word "No!".

Allow that "No!" to shatter those previous negative images like a sheet of glass, and notice that it reveals the long-term, positive consequences of achieving your goal. Make this experience vivid and compelling. Add more and more details to what you can see, hear and feel until it feels like it's actually happening right now and you can feel the excitement and happiness in your body. Notice the positive impacts this has had in every area of your life, professionally, socially, privately, intimately. Spend long enough in this moment for it to feel real.

Open your eyes and distract yourself for a moment. Notice something happening outside yourself, or remember something random and abstract. This prevents the process looping on itself, since we are about to repeat this process several times.

Do this process five to 10 times, getting faster and faster, until your conscious mind can barely keep up, and your unconscious mind takes over.

Exercise: pain and pleasure?

Any time you spot yourself about to engage in an activity that is not in alignment with your goals, ask yourself "what is the pain and pleasure I am focused on right now?" Self-awareness and self-honesty are an important part of achieving your goals. Then use the re-patterning exercise to re-programme your behaviour.

Life Vision

Not only do we get Push and Pull competition between the motivation to achieve our longer-term goals (e.g. body transformation), and our short-term desires for instant, easily accessible pleasure (e.g. the TV and pizza), we can also get Push and Pull competition between the other goals we have in life. After all, achieving a physical transformation isn't the only thing that's important to you. You also have career goals, financial goals, relationship goals, recreational goals and so on, each of which have Push and Pull motivational forces of their own, all competing for your time, focus, and energy throughout the day.

I see a lot of people getting stuck in focusing all their time, effort and energy on just one aspect of their life, for example, their career. Everything else gets neglected, and inevitably deteriorates.

At this point one of two things usually happens. Either they ignore all the symptoms and tell themselves "I'll deal with it later, when I've got time, after I've..." and continue to push harder in their career, perhaps even using work as an anaesthetic to distract themselves from the pain in other areas of their life. They may indeed achieve impressive feats in their career, but at some point something breaks. Their marriage breaks down, they fall severely ill, and then all of a sudden all their achievements in their career don't count for much. All the status and money suddenly seem less important when you've lost the person you love, or when you're in hospital fighting for your life.

The other common outcome is that at some point one of these other areas deteriorates so much, and the pain (Push motivation) in that area becomes so severe that they panic, drop what they were doing and focus all their energy on this area instead, to the detriment of everything else. They end up in a pattern of firefighting, constantly changing direction, trying to patch up the biggest pain in their life, going around in circles but never getting any nearer to the life they want to live.

The solution is to recognise that in fact, these goals are not in competition with each other, but are all interdependent - equally important parts of a bigger picture. If you neglect any of these areas for long enough, eventually the consequences will spill out into the other parts of your life. In order for you to live a truly happy and fulfilling life, every one of these areas needs consistent time, effort and energy.

Achieving a sustainable body transformation becomes harder if you feel stuck and helpless in your career or relationship. Pursuing your career ambitions becomes much harder if you are in a destructive relationship. Finding, or maintaining a happy, loving, fulfilling relationship is so much harder if you feel insecure about your body, feel self-conscious, or suffer low self-esteem.

This does not mean that you cannot achieve a body transformation until everything else is perfect in your life. It means that when you feel stuck, helpless and unhappy, those emotions will leak out in symptoms and coping mechanisms that are highly likely to sabotage your goals. It also means that when you lack clarity and direction, your daily actions tend to be reactive, inconsistent, and typically Away From rather than Towards orientated.

Accepting full accountability for your stock in life, setting exciting goals, and exercising your personal power to chase those goals is extraordinarily empowering and liberating. Everything else becomes easier when you feel in control of yourself and your life, and that you are shaping your destiny.

You need to have a clearly-defined, exciting body trans-formation goal, but you also need to know where that fits in the big picture of your life. You need to have an all-encompassing vision for your life that includes the things that matter to you the most, such as health, wealth and love, and you need to be able to see how your physical goal fits into and contributes to that big picture: your Life Vision. This Life Vision encompasses not only the goals you will achieve and acquire – the destination so to speak - but also the journey, *how* you live your life and your experience of life along the way.

Each of these areas of your Life Vision need consis-tent time, energy, and action to maintain their existing condition, let alone move forward. So we need to plan a schedule that supports that.

Once you have designed your Life Vision, you will create what is essentially a business plan for your life that breaks down each of these goals into manageable steps, and ultimately into a schedule you follow every day. This way your goals will work together to create an exciting, passionate life that makes you truly happy. This is how you create sustainable long-term and successful goals.

When you have a truly exciting Life Vision, and a high-quality plan and schedule for achieving it, you can recognise how every single activity is an important and integral part of creating that Life Vision. This is particularly important for those activities that used to seem boring, insignificant or mundane in the past.

When you can associate those small, yet vital steps with the ultimate achievement of your Life Vision and a happy, exciting, and passionate life, boredom gets replaced with passion, and you will achieve that critical ingredient of success – consistency.

Exercise: Life Vision

Decide on the key areas of your life that matter to you the most. These are entirely your choice, but the most common areas include:

- » Career goals
- » Financial goals
- » Relationship goals, which you may choose to subdivide into:
    - » Intimate relationship
    - » Family
    - » Friends
- » Physical goals
- » Recreational goals
- » Spiritual, or mindset goals

Write down your goals in each of these areas. Once again, be sure to include the emotions you want to feel more of, and the reasons *why* you want these things. Repeat this exercise once a week. Over time you will update, improve, and evolve your Life Vision as you learn more about yourself, the world, and what you *really* want. Your Life Vision is also likely to grow as you break through limiting beliefs that held you back in the past.

Read your Life Vision goals every single day.

Exercise: Assess in context

Assess all your activities, habits and behaviours in the context of your Life Vision. Identify when you are engaged in activities that do not contribute to your Life Vision (e.g. mindlessly scrolling through social media). Time is the one thing you can never make back. Use it wisely.

Scheduling

A goal will never become a reality until you plan and schedule it. It's very common for some people to write down their goals, and to immediately feel comfortable – to the point where they don't feel any pressure to take any further action: the very yo-yo pattern we discussed earlier. If you have done this yourself I would suggest that that feeling of comfort immediately after finishing a goal-setting exercise is one of your triggers for self-sabotage, and that you run the re-patterning exercise on it.

Immediately after finishing a goal-setting session, do something that commits you to continuing the momentum. For example, you could immediately invest money in it, or book a meeting or appointment.

Beyond this it is critical you create a plan for the accomplishment of your goal, and schedule the activities necessary. All too often people have vague ideas of "I'll do it when I have time" and then wonder why they don't get results. Imagine if Tom Watson had attempted to build his vision for IBM by keeping his schedule, lifestyle, and habits the same and fit the activities for building the company around *"when he had time"*. It would never have worked. And yet that is how some people run their lives and then are surprised when 15 years later nothing has changed!

We need to create a plan for building your Life Vision. If your Life Vision is big and bold then the plan will also need to be big and detailed. This can be overwhelming at first so let's start small, take it one goal at a time and chunk each one down.

Chunking

In 1985 Joe Simpson and Simon Yates successfully made the first ascent of the Siula Grande in the Peruvian Andes. During the descent, Joe fell and broke his leg, his shin bone splitting the knee. Simon Yates took it upon himself to lower Joe down most of the mountain. During this rescue a turn of events resulted in Joe falling into a crevasse and becoming separated from Simon.

In spite of his terrible injuries, Joe lowered himself further into the crevasse and managed to find a way out. Suffering from hypothermia and dehydration, he still had to cross a glacier unroped and then the moraines (the rock fields created by glaciers). He crawled and hobbled in perpetual pain for three and half days, all the way back to Base Camp, finding Simon just hours before they were due to leave.

In his book *Touching the Void* Joe mentions that when he considered the task that faced him it felt insurmountable. His strategy was to break it up into small steps: he focussed exclusively on a target 100m away and set a time limit for reaching it. When he reached it he would then set the next target, and so on.

This is exactly how we need to approach the goals within our Life Vision.

Set Intermediate Goals

Let's start with your physical goal. If you have set yourself a goal for 12 months' time, where do you need to be at in six, three, and then one month? Write these intermediate goals down now. These targets may move or need adjusting as you gain feedback along the way and learn more about yourself and your goal. Joe Simpson didn't always hit the time deadlines he set himself. It's having the target, and doing everything you can to hit it that matters.

Once you have your one-month goal, set yourself a daily and weekly schedule for accomplishing it. With regards to your physical goal I suggest you schedule the following activities:

> » The days and times for each of your workouts

> » What you are going to eat every day and when. This needs to be planned at least one day in advance; if you make last minute food decisions you are guaranteed to go off plan.

> » What food you need to buy, where from and when

> » Back-up options for when you get bored

> » Contingency plans for when something goes wrong

> » Also prepare for meals out, and decide what types of food and drink choices you will make.

Actually write these tasks in your diary. Long-term success is significantly greater when people schedule these tasks rather than making mental notes of when they would like to get them done.

Life Vision Planning

Make a commitment to gradually fill in the rest of your plan for your Life Vision. I got you to plan your physical goal first, as I am assuming that is high on your priority list.

Next, make a list of each of your remaining goals in the order in which you would like to tackle them. All that matters is that you set the game up to win. Some people prefer to schedule the goals that are the easiest to plan, so they get a sense of progress and momentum. Others prefer to schedule goals that require a bigger, more detailed plan first (a business or career goal for example), since this gives them a strong sense of motivation and drive.

Commit to planning and scheduling at least one goal per week. Make sure you get a clear sense of how these different goals will work alongside each other, work together, and support each other towards your Life Vision. By the end of the process you should have a clear idea of how you are going to live your life. This should fill you with excitement because you can clearly see your outcome, and your purpose at the end of it all.

Mental Recovery and Downtime

One more note on building your plan. Make sure you schedule mental recovery and downtime into each day and each week. Some people, particularly perfectionists, can find it tempting to think that they can get more done in the short term by blasting through without taking any breaks. This may work for a few days, or a few weeks, but it is not sustainable. It is true that you can work much longer and harder when you love what you do. Most people who reach burn out do so in jobs that feel frustrating or out of their control.

However, even if you love what you do, recovery is extremely important for mental and physical health. You will also find that, ironically, your productivity will increase when you regularly schedule time for your mind and body to reset. Your energy and ability to focus will improve dramatically.

The other significant benefit is that when you schedule this balance, your unconscious mind won't force you to take time out.

Loss of concentration, daydreaming mid task, compulsive or addictive behaviours such as binge eating and smoking are all examples of common symptoms when someone hasn't given their mind and body the time it needs to switch off.

It is your brain's way of saying "Hey dummy! I need a break!"

Find the schedule of downtime that is appropriate for you. Some people respond really well by having a 45-minute walk at the end of the day. Other people do well scheduling one or two meditation breaks of 10-20 minutes each day. This will be challenging to schedule for many people, such as parents of young babies, but if you put your mind to it you will be able to find a way to achieve some level of consistency.

The most important thing is that this downtime is 100% brain off, no work, phones, or social media etc. You must allow your mind to switch off and unwind fully.

I also recommend most people take one day per week (often a Sunday) that involves no work or formal exercise.

Summary

All humans are motivated by two forces: pain and pleasure. We call the pain we wish to avoid Push motivation, and the pleasure we are drawn towards Pull motivation. These forces apply not only to the big goals in your life (such as transforming your body), but all the small decisions you make as well (such as deciding to go out with friends or stay in).

Towards and Away From thinking underpins any area of personal change. If you want to improve an area of your life you *must* identify what you want to add or move towards, instead of what you want to reduce, eliminate, escape, or move away from. Wanting to *lose weight* so that you can *feel less self-conscious*, in the hope that you suffer from *less rejection,* are all examples of Away From thinking. Wanting to build a healthy body with sexy curves, with extraordinary well-being and vitality, so that you can experience more energy and confidence in all aspects of your life are examples of Towards thinking.

In addition to the SMART acronym, goals must be stated in Towards language, in the present tense, be genuinely exciting, identify the emotions of *why* this goal is important to you, and incorporate a range to allow flexibility.

People yo-yo because they stop focusing on the long-term pain and pleasure associated with transforming their body, and start focusing on the easier, short-term pain and pleasure. To establish the consistency necessary for a successful body transformation you must attach your long-term pain and pleasure associated with your goals to those specific moments when you used to sabotage yourself. Re-patterning allows you to programme your unconscious mind to do this automatically.

It is critical to understand how your body goals fit into the big picture context of your life, and that you intentionally work towards a life that both makes you truly happy and fulfilled, and is congruent with your body goals. You must design and revisit your Life Vision regularly to maintain long-term motivation for your body goals. Your body affects your life, and your life affects your body.

Chapter 2

Mental Rehearsal and Identity

What You Will Learn

» Why willpower is unreliable as a way to keep yourself on track.

» One of the biggest causes for self-sabotage, and why some behaviours may feel out of your control.

» How your sense of identity controls your behaviour, and your ultimate success.

» How your identity is created and how to create a sense of identity at the unconscious level to support your goals.

» How to programme your unconscious mind so you automatically think, feel, and behave in ways that support your body transformation and enhance motivation, tenacity, consistency, and passion.

Mental Rehearsal

Mental rehearsal is a technique commonly used in the sporting and athletic world. When an athlete mentally rehearses performing their sport exactly the way they want, it makes those specific skills and behaviours more automatic. The effect and power of mental rehearsal, which has been well researched and documented, is that it:

» improves mental control

» improves physical performance

» helps to make behaviours and skills automatic

» increases motivation

» encourages setting higher goals

» improves adherence to training

Mental rehearsal works in large part because the unconscious mind cannot tell the difference between what is real and what is vividly imagined. For example, if you sit there and will your heart rate to go faster, you probably find that you can't do it. But if you vividly imagine yourself in a dark alley with a stranger approaching you with a knife, and you really imagine all the details about what you can see, hear and feel, then your heart starts to beat faster, your breathing rate goes up, your palms start to sweat and so on. Your mind and body respond in the same way whether it's happening for real or just being imagined. Your unconscious mind cannot tell the difference between reality and imagination.

When an athlete mentally rehearses a particular sporting skill, reaction, or outcome, they are strengthening the sequence of messages in their nervous system, which in turn reinforces those skills and makes them more automatic.

Unfortunately, many people have accidentally learnt how to use mental rehearsal to install precisely the behaviours they want to avoid.

A common example I come across all the time is where people mentally rehearse cravings and binge eating. Perhaps they have been invited to a party at the weekend and they are worried about "breaking their diet". Since they are worried about it they think about it. They vividly imagine the behaviour they don't want to do.

(Remember our "don't think of a black cat" demonstration? The brain doesn't know how not to do something.)

They imagine all the food that will be on display. They imagine the cupcakes covered in icing in vivid detail. They imagine what they look like and what they smell like. They imagine what it feels like to scoop some of that icing onto their finger. They imagine what it feels and tastes like to suck the icing off their finger and swallow it. They create a vivid multisensory experience of bingeing!

When they get to the party they are on high alert for all the temptations. Inevitably they find them, stare at them and go through the whole process again.

Then they use their willpower to try to resist bingeing! But of course, willpower is a conscious activity, and you can't stay consciously focused on resisting the whole time - it's exhausting. So eventually the unconscious mind takes over and carries out the automatic programme they have pre-installed. They used mental rehearsal to pre-install bingeing, so of course that's what happens!

Your imagination dominates your will.

Recall how I mentioned that Towards and Away From language permeates everything we do, and Away From language frequently shows up when people are stuck with a problem. This is a perfect example.

What this person *really* wants has nothing to do with what they don't want. If we drill down and ask them what they do want they may say, "To show my friends how much I love them, laugh, reminisce, find out what's new with them, update them on what I've been doing, feel excited, feel love, feel confident".

After all, what does somebody who maintains a slim, fit, and healthy figure, and who has no issues with binge eating, think about when they are at a party? They focus precisely on what they *do* want. Worrying about "not bingeing" doesn't even cross their mind.

To reiterate: your unconscious mind doesn't know the difference between reality and imagination, so if you've simply *imagined* things going wrong, then you are effectively using mental rehearsal to programme your unconscious mind to fail.

Furthermore, if you've been in the habit of reminding yourself of unpleasant memories or experiences over and over in your mind, as far as your nervous system is concerned that is literally like reliving them again. As a consequence, you are adding more and more examples of that type of reference experience to the storage banks in your brain. All of this will have an influence on how your brain spontaneously reacts and behaves in the future.

What does this mean for you? Whether you are remembering things that you have labelled as failures in the past, or imagine yourself failing in the future, you are using mental rehearsal to programme failure into your unconscious mind.

Identity

Mental rehearsal works on two levels: firstly it installs and strengthens specific behaviours. An athlete will mentally rehearse specific skills. Our dieter at the party can either mentally rehearse binge eating, or mentally rehearse being the life and soul of the party, making jokes, feeling confident, and really connecting with their friends.

Secondly, mental rehearsal will serve to design and reinforce the sense of identity you hold at the unconscious level.

An athlete will imagine themselves a winner, possessed of talent, hard work, desire, dedication, determination, tenacity, and a willingness to do whatever it takes. They condition themselves to think and feel this way through practice and repetition. Remember Mohammad Ali and his mantra "I am the greatest!"

Your identity – your sense of self – forms the blueprint your unconscious mind uses to guide your decisions and behaviour. When you think of yourself and your body, what are the first thoughts, images, or words that come to mind? Do you think of yourself as someone who struggles with their body, with low self-esteem, and no self-discipline? If so then it's inevitable that you'll sabotage yourself, mindlessly eat, and skip workouts, because those behaviours are congruent with that identity.

Your Unconscious Identity is a set of beliefs about who you really are. This identity - like all beliefs - is a choice. The identity you carry around with you now is simply a set of generalisations, assumptions, and guesses, which you can change if they are not serving you. Mental rehearsal is how you do that.

You must think of yourself as already being the person you will become once you achieve your ideal weight and body shape. What qualities, attributes, and behaviours do you have? How do you live your life? What choices do you make? What values and rules do you live by? How do you spend your time?

Imagine yourself as already being that way - just like Tom Watson did with IBM – and that you simply need to allow more time for your physiology - your health and body shape - to catch up.

An athlete who gets an injury and is in rehab may lose all physical conditioning. Even so, they still see themselves as an athlete - and they approach their rehab with the same focus and dedication. In time their physiology catches up, and their physical image matches their internal image.

See yourself as already a slim, toned, healthy person, with the mindset, lifestyle, and behaviours to match. You are telling your unconscious mind you are different now, you have changed. You are installing a new blueprint with a completely new set of instructions and you will find yourself automatically and spontaneously living your life in a way that supports your goals.

Doing this is going to take some practice and repetition. We have to recondition your mind to project new images, new dialogue, and a new identity to yourself until it becomes second nature.

If you've been overweight for a while, or if you've previously struggled to change your body shape, when you look at your past what do you notice? How long you've been overweight and how difficult it's been. Whenever you think about your body, or dieting or weight loss, you instantly refer to these images, thoughts and feelings, simply because they are familiar and easy to access. They are reinforced and multiplied.

The mind favours familiarity and the path of least resistance. When you imagine the future, the easiest images to create are ones you already have experience of. So you simply project those same images into the future and inevitably keep yourself stuck in the same predictable pattern.

The chances are that you've been doing this without even realising it, and if that's the case, you are going to think of yourself as an overweight person, who struggles to lose weight. How do you think this is going to affect your behaviour and your chances of success in the future? Of course, you'll think "what's the point?".

You can change all this, in an instant. You need to create positive, successful reference experiences that dominate and overwhelm the old ones. Your overriding image of yourself - your default reference point - needs to be that of a healthy, fit, motivated and powerful you who can achieve anything.

Whenever you think of yourself, food, exercise or fat loss, these successful thoughts and images need to overwhelm any negative ones. This way, when your brain thinks, "what normally happens here?" it will instantly be reminded of lots of successful experiences of you being lean, fit, active and consistently making healthy choices. Whether these successful experiences were real or imagined, your unconscious won't know the difference and will expect success in the future, spontaneously drawing you towards it.

Do The Work

"Thinking is the hardest work there is, which is the probably reason why so few engage in it."

Henry Ford

"There is no expedient to which a man will not go to avoid the real labour of thinking."

Thomas Edison

Learning to run your brain with mental rehearsal gives you total control over your life, but unfortunately, most people will do anything to avoid the effort it takes to develop this skill. After all, it's a lot easier to just start a new diet, right? That's much more exciting!

If you want a successful physical transformation, mental rehearsal is a skill you must develop and use. And just like any other skill, you must exercise that mental muscle for it to get stronger. It may feel weird to begin with. This is normal and is a good sign, because it means it is different!

Mental rehearsal is an incredibly powerful technique and when used consistently, it allows you to programme those behaviours that will lead you to success.

Guided Mental Rehearsal

I'm going to describe a typical mental rehearsal session to you in the same way that I would if I were in the room with you. Take your time reading this section to allow yourself to see, hear and feel the details I describe in vivid detail.

Transport yourself into the future to a time and place where you've already achieved your goals for your body, your fitness and your health. As you find yourself travelling forwards through time to this date, notice the image of the totally new you standing proudly in front of you: a fit, healthy, confident, vibrant you. Notice this image becoming more and more real with each passing moment. In the same way that you can look at another person and tell that they ooze health, fitness and confidence, notice how this image of you radiates the qualities you would like to have more of.

Perhaps you would like to add more confidence. So pour more and more confidence into that you standing there. Allow your unconscious mind to draw on times when you've been confident in the past, as well as from inspirational examples of confident people you admire.

Notice how that you changes when you have access to all that confidence whenever you need it. Notice how your posture changes, how your facial expression changes, how you carry yourself differently, how you interact with others differently, how your voice volume and tonality changes.

And then do the same thing with any other qualities you'd like more of. Perhaps energy, enthusiasm, passion, determination, tenacity, peace or love for yourself.

Notice the fantastic body shape that you've created for yourself. See the contours of your body, defined by the shape of your muscles. Notice how lean and fit you are. See how much energy, vigour and vitality your movements have during your workouts. See how differently you move, even during normal daily activity. Notice the healthy glow to your complexion, admire that confident spring in your step, and see this new you interacting in new ways that delight you.

I don't know if this image is already life-size as you look at it, or whether it gradually becomes the same height as you the more you marvel and admire it, but you can notice how bright and vibrant the colours become, and perhaps you can even notice the whole image sizzling and glowing with its energy and radiance. As the power of that image continues to grow, add a soundtrack. Let that creative part of you choose one piece of music that fills you with confidence and power and stands out as being the most powerful, the most useful or the most appropriate.

Take the time to revel in the beauty of this image and add anything that makes it even better. Once you can really feel the appeal of this new fit, healthy, vibrant you, step inside this image and become this new you. Feel how amazing it is to be lean, fit and healthy. You've made such a dramatic change to your body and your health that other people ask you how you've done it. Notice how you hold yourself differently now that you are so fit and healthy. Notice what it's like standing in front of the mirror and seeing how fit and firm your body looks. Look how much energy you have and how it feels to walk around in this fit, strong, healthy, vibrant body. Notice the reactions of other people in your life and the impact this change has had in every area of your life: socially, at home, privately, even at work. Feel how much your confidence and your self-esteem have surged and how that affects every other area of your life. Notice what you say to yourself in your mind: I'm so proud of myself for having been so consistent and I'm so grateful now that I can thoroughly enjoy being so fit and healthy. I love the fact that I am in total control of my life, my eating habits and my body, I'm so excited by the fact that I now love exercising and the feeling of energy and vitality that it gives me, the way it has transformed my body, my self-esteem and my confidence. Add any other internal dialogue that really hits the spot for you and makes you feel even better. Notice how thinking, feeling and *being* this way helps you to impact and improve *other* people's lives, especially those of the important people around you.

Spend some time moving around in your strong, fit, energetic, healthy body. Notice what it feels like during normal daily movements. Then feel how amazing it feels totally dominating a high intensity workout.

Also notice the healthy habits that have become a natural part of who you are and what you do every day, such as exercising regularly and loving it. Notice what it's like working out now you've achieved such incredible improvements in your fitness and strength. And also notice how eating healthily is a normal, natural part of your daily routine. Making healthy, appropriate food choices is easy; it has become a natural and permanent way of being for you.

As you continue to notice what you can see, what you can hear and what you can feel now that you have successfully and permanently achieved your body and health goals, look back at the lifestyle that has led you to this point. Notice how you've behaved, your lifestyle and the milestones that have led you to achieve such great success. Notice how you've made steady progress by applying yourself every day, every week. Enjoy how your routine and lifestyle have evolved into what is now an easy, normal, natural way of living for you. Things that seemed daunting and challenging before are now so simple: social environments, food shopping, meal prep, meal timings, time management and so on are all so easy to handle because you've done it hundreds of times. Life is so much more fun and rewarding now you've stuck to your guns and applied yourself to something that really matters to you. As you look back at your journey, notice those obstacles you faced, the challenges that crop up in the pursuit of any worthwhile goal. Notice how you overcame them and how you learnt from them.

Spend a few more moments enjoying life in your fit, healthy, energetic body, and then travel back to the present, bringing with you this wonderful experience and new way of being, and look out at this new future that you have created for yourself. See that journey stretching out in front of you, and recognise that this is the way things are going to be from now on.

Raise Your Standards

Your life will not get better until *you* get better. To succeed in any transformation programme, you will need to raise your standards in terms of what you expect from yourself: how you think, and how you behave. You do that by designing your Unconscious Identity- that image you have of yourself in your head and the type of person you think you are. Then if you're ever tempted to go off track, you'll say to yourself "No! This isn't me, I'm better than this".

You need to start in the future - just like Tom Watson. You need to start with a clear and vivid vision of yourself as already a slim, lean, fit individual and then live your life in the present in a way that reflects that new identity.

Get Detailed

To get the greatest benefit out of your mental rehearsal sessions, make sure you make them as vivid and multi-sensory as possible. Add lots of details to what you can see, hear, and feel. Make the images big, bright, detailed, vibrant, colourful, moving images. Make the sounds clear and crisp and just the right volume for maximum impact. Feel all the relevant kinaesthetic details that make the experience even more powerful, increase the feelings of energy and strength, and notice how it feels when you have that sense of complete confidence and pride in yourself.

Some people are able to create vivid and powerful experiences during mental rehearsal right away. Others need a little more practice. It doesn't matter what your starting point is. This is a very important skill that will continue to improve with practice, so make sure you schedule time to develop it.

Your Default Reference Point

The greater the degree of stress we are under, the more we tend to react automatically without thinking.

This new identity needs to become the dominant opinion you have of yourself. It needs to become your default reference point – an automatic response whether you are in a good mood and relaxed, or whether you are put into a stressful situation.

Your new identity needs to be vivid and complete enough to be immediately accessible by your unconscious mind. You will need to keep practising mental rehearsal to maintain this condition, and building yourself from the inside out in this manner should become a lifelong habit.

When, How Frequently and For How Long?

In order for this new identity and these new experiences to become your default reference point and completely dominate any old negative ones from the past, how often should you do your mental rehearsal sessions?

I want you to do your mental rehearsal exercise *at least* once a day, but to begin with you may need to do it more frequently to ensure you overwrite the old rubbish.

Also, at any point throughout the day, if you ever notice yourself about to remember any disappointments from the past or imagine failure in the future, instantly stop, and replace those images with successful ones from your mental rehearsal sessions. And the same goes for your internal language as well as your internal images. So if you ever notice yourself saying negative or defeatist things to yourself, immediately replace them with empowering, uplifting words, delivered with certainty and congruence.

Take as long as you need to make each mental rehearsal feel powerful and compelling. At first this will probably take you anywhere between five and 20 minutes. With practice you'll speed up and will eventually be able to fully immerse yourself in it in seconds - but don't sell yourself short. The more frequently and the more thoroughly you do this exercise the more effective it will be. This is not a one hit wonder. We are conditioning ourselves every day, so make sure that you make the time to do this every day. It doesn't take long, but the return you get from it is extraordinary.

Back It Up With Action

You need to back up your Unconscious Identity with action. It is very important to reinforce your internal with your external reality so you feel congruent and aligned. Otherwise it's like making promises to yourself and repeatedly breaking them - it destroys your integrity, self-confidence, and self-belief. That doesn't mean you're never allowed to make mistakes, it means you do what you say you will do.

So this process is constantly being reinforced and updated:

» Design your identity - your ideal image of your ideal self. If you want to achieve all you set out to achieve, what type of person do you need to become? What qualities, skills, attributes, and behaviours do you need to develop and nurture?

» Use mental rehearsal to communicate that identity, and the behaviours that go along with it to your unconscious mind. See, hear, and feel yourself being the type of person you want to be

» Refer to that image regularly throughout the day and use it to guide your behaviour

» Repeatedly check if your current thoughts, focus, and behaviour match that image, and if not, make the necessary adjustments

» Update your Unconscious Identity as you grow, learn and evolve

» Repeat

Summary of Steps for Mental Rehearsal

1: **Comfort and privacy**: get yourself in a comfortable sitting or reclining position where you can safely close your eyes and remain undisturbed for 10 minutes. Switch off your phone and other distractions.

2: **Disassociated**: imagine seeing yourself from a third person's perspective once you have already achieved your goal. Use both your eyes and ears. Notice your physique and how you move. See yourself in vivid detail as looking, feeling and behaving exactly the way you want to be. Make this image exciting and compelling. Also hear yourself speak in exactly the way you want. Add a soundtrack if you like; perhaps uplifting commentary, or uplifting music.

Add qualities and resources you would like to see more of in yourself and amplify them: such as confidence, calmness, tenacity and so on, always there - available whenever you want and need them.

Things to think about: Who are you now? What kind of person have you become? What qualities do you have more of? How do you act and conduct yourself from day to day, moment to moment? How do you respond to what you used to perceive as stress? How do you respond when you're really busy? Ensure that your identity and behaviour are congruent with being fit, healthy and in the best shape of your life.

3: **Associated**: once you can see and hear yourself looking, behaving, and being exactly the way you want, step inside that image so that you become that image and feel what it feels like from the inside. Don't step inside the image until the disassociated image looks exactly as you want it to. Make it right from a third person's perspective first, then step inside it. Add lots of details to the experience so that it feels as though it is actually happening right now. When you first do this, it might take a bit more time and focus, but with practice you'll soon be able to create a vivid and compelling experience, and each time you do it you'll be able to recreate it more and more quickly. Make it a multi-sensory experience, so include lots of details in what you can see, what you can hear and what you can feel (visual, auditory and kinaesthetic). Also add empowering internal dialogue ("I am amazing, I can do anything"). Notice what it feels like to walk, talk and move in this body. Notice how it feels to BE this way all day every day. What do you do each day? Who do you spend time with? What is your lifestyle like? Notice the types of decisions and choices you make, and feel how life enhancing and fulfilling it feels to consistently make choices that are in alignment with your life goals.

Note: With practice you will be able to make Steps Two and Three more and more detailed and vivid. Over time add to the experiences: more situations, environments, behaviours and qualities.

4: **Look back at the journey**: having already achieved your goal, look back at the journey and the lifestyle that has led you to this point. Notice the milestones you hit along the way, the breakthrough moments. Notice obstacles and how you overcame them. Notice how every moment of every day your thoughts, decisions and actions were designed in the mould of your new identity, and how this became a natural habit for you, every day, every week, every month. Notice how exciting the journey has been. Look back with pride.

5: **Bring into the present**: float back to the present moment, bringing with you that new identity and lifestyle so that it naturally feels like this is who you are and what you do every day. Look into the future and know that this is how you will live your life from now on.

Summary

Mental rehearsal programmes your unconscious mind. It makes behaviours more automatic, reinforces beliefs, increases motivation, and programmes your unconsciously held sense of identity.

Your unconscious mind cannot tell the difference between a real experience and something that is vividly imagined. Your unconsciously-held sense of identity dictates your behaviour, choices, and your ultimate destiny.

To succeed in transforming your body forever, you must vividly imagine yourself already being the way you want to be, not just physically, but mentally and emotionally as well, with the mindset, confidence, beliefs, attitude, and application of someone who is already slim, fit, and healthy.

People often self-sabotage, as in the example of binge eating, simply because they spend so much time worrying about what they hope won't happen. They use mental rehearsal to programme the very behaviour they want to avoid.

Mental rehearsal should include lots of details about what you can *see,* what you can *hear,* and what you can *feel*. It should be practised until it becomes your default reference point.

Having programmed your Unconscious Identity, and the behaviours to match, you must back up this sense of identity with action. Actually do what you have just communicated to your unconscious mind that you will do.

3 Believe

What You Will Learn

» How beliefs dictate whether you will succeed or fail in your body transformation.

» How beliefs are created and strengthened.

» How people learn to doubt themselves and their abilities.

» How the brain makes generalisations that become mistaken as the truth.

» How people develop learned help-lessness – a mental poison that guarantees failure.

» How beliefs are destroyed and replaced: how to identify the limiting beliefs that used to hold you back from the body you want, and get rid of them forever.

» How to create extraordinary self-belief that propels you towards the body you want, and a lifetime of health and vitality.

Beliefs

"What if I'm just meant to be overweight?"

Sadly, I hear this all the time. Most of these people are smart and well educated but have a terrible relationship with themselves and food, which leads to desperate thoughts and poor decisions.

"What if I am meant to be overweight...I'm desperate to lose weight, but I have always been fat, and tried and failed on every diet."

This is a fear that ironically is keeping them overweight.

Beliefs are the unconscious filters through which we process information and make decisions. They influence our perception of life, our experience of life, and our destiny. They control the journey, *and* the destination.

When aligned and used effectively, beliefs can give you purpose, direction, tenacity, resilience, the drive to succeed and the faith that you *will* succeed.

On the other hand, limiting beliefs can be among the most destructive forces in your life, holding you back, sabotaging your progress, and causing doubt, helplessness, even depression.

If you don't believe to your very core that you will succeed, then at some point you'll ask yourself "what's the point?" and if you don't have an immediate and powerful response to that question you'll sabotage your progress.

Placebo

Most people are familiar with the placebo effect. When a patient expects to recover, this has a profound effect on their actual recovery. If a patient is administered a placebo via injection, it has been discovered that the placebo effect is greater than if it is administered via a pill, simply because injections are associated with more powerful drugs, and the patient expects a more profound response. This expectation translates into a more pronounced physiological recovery.

The placebo effect also works in reverse via the nocebo effect. In other words, symptoms, illness and disease can be induced simply via the expectation of that outcome.

This isn't just relevant in disease and medicine, it permeates everything you do. The results you get in business, relationships, or weight loss are highly dependent on your beliefs in those areas.

Beliefs and Weight Loss

Consider someone embarking on a weight loss programme who has absolute certainty that the programme works and will work for them. They apply themselves fully. They may make mistakes and have setbacks, but they know with absolute certainty that they are on the right track and as a consequence they remain committed and resilient. They will get good results, which provide them with stronger evidence of their capabilities, and the effectiveness of the programme. This in turn further reinforces the belief that they can do it.

So these three phases:

1. Belief

2. Commitment and Application

3. Results and Evidence, and then back to Belief become a cycle that gets stronger and stronger as it fuels itself.

Now consider someone who embarks on the same weight loss programme, but this person has doubts and fears about their own capabilities. They have tried to lose weight in the past and only ended up heavier, and they are now worried that maybe they're just meant to be this way. As a consequence, part of them is already thinking *"what's the point?"* They *try,* but inevitably their commitment and application suffers. Their poor or variable results provide them with evidence of their limitations, which further reinforces the belief that "I can't do it; maybe I'm just meant to be this way".

This person is caught in a very different cycle:

1. Self-doubt

2. Trying and struggling

3. Underperforming, poor results, and evidence of their limitations, then back to even more self-doubt.

What Comes First?

In both these examples, the *belief* starts the whole process off and dictates the ultimate outcome. Even if someone starts with what some may consider to be a *realistic* attitude such as "I hope this works, let's see what happens", they will get very different results to someone who starts with the attitude of "I know I will make this work. Whatever happens, I will find a way".

Unfortunately, many people develop debilitating limiting beliefs that sabotage any attempt they subsequently make to lose weight.

A very common example might be as follows: they grew up in an unhealthy environment, tried to lose weight on a low-calorie diet, and lost weight but hammered their metabolism in the process, ending up putting the weight back on with interest. Then they tried low fat diets, but this resulted in hormone dysfunction, as fat is essential for hormonal health, and after a brief period of weight loss they rebounded again.

Next they tried low carb diets, but soon hit a plateau, suffered horrendous cravings for carbs and sugar, and kept breaking their diet. By this point, in addition to wondering "why is this so hard?" and "why can't I do it?" they are also questioning their will power.

Then maybe they stumble across a really sensible diet but get barely any results for several weeks and give up. What they didn't realise is that it will take a while to repair the damage caused by all the unhealthy and extreme dieting, and that after a period of recovering their internal health, their body would have started dropping fat effectively, if only they had remained patient and consistent.

From their perspective, all the evidence points to the fact (belief) that they're just meant to be overweight. In fact they have simply tried one flawed approach after another, and have accumulated a wealth of reference experiences that they have labelled as failure and evidence that "I can't do it".

The process often goes further and gets worse:

Part of them starts to ask the question, "what if I'm just meant to be overweight?"

They desperately hope this isn't the case, but they're terrified it might be true. If they threw themselves into a fat loss programme, tried their hardest to make it work, but "failed", that would "prove" their fears to be true. So to protect themselves from proving they can't do it they sabotage themselves, hold something back, and don't commit 100%. At least that way they can fall back on the excuse "I didn't give it my all. Next time I'll give it everything".

Of course, they never really do give it everything because what if they failed?

This pattern is extremely common, and people are often completely unaware that they are doing it.

With the correct approach, this person can absolutely recover their health, achieve a healthy weight, build a lean, fit, healthy body, and keep it for the rest of their life. It's basic physiology. But for that to happen they must destroy their old limiting beliefs and replace them with new, empowering beliefs.

Psychologist and author of *Learned Optimism,* Martin Seligman has identified the patterns of belief that cause us to feel helpless. They are:

» **Permanence**: believing in the permanence of a problem – "I'll always be overweight".

» **Pervasiveness**: believing in the pervasiveness of a problem. Allowing a problem to dominate so much in your life that it feels like your life is the problem. "I can't lose weight because I'm unhappy, but being overweight makes me unhappy in every area of my life".

» **Personal**: believing in the personal nature of a problem. Making the problem a part of your identity – "It's just who I am".

These beliefs are not facts. They were incorrect assumptions based on very limited data that have become generalised and mistaken for reality.

One of the fundamental principles of excellence is the awareness that our beliefs are a choice. They are not something you have, are given, or that happen to you. Beliefs are something you *do*.

Let's explore how this happens, the structure of beliefs, and how they are maintained.

The Structure of Beliefs - Filtering

Your brain makes rapid generalisations. This is useful because it means you can make decisions very quickly without having to analyse and assess every situation. However, it can be a double-edged sword because we can attach meanings to events that are not useful.

For example, does failing to achieve and maintain a body transformation on a low-calorie juice diet mean that you're just meant to be overweight, or does it just mean that low calorie juice diets are utterly ridiculous, harmful, and unsustainable?

Beliefs are supported by a process called filtering. When you buy a new car, all of a sudden you notice that car everywhere you go. Your brain has been put on high alert to notice that car. You are filtering *in* certain information. We also filter things out. Perhaps you are looking for a particular item in the supermarket, but you can't see it. The manufacturer has changed the packaging, so even though the product is right there in front of you, because you're filtering for a particular colour and design, you don't see it.

Men do this all the time. They want food and go to the fridge, look, do not find anything and then complain to their wife that there is no food in the house. She goes to the fridge and pulls out three different food choices! I am frequently guilty of this one!

We are constantly filtering our experience. Everyone is deleting, distorting, and generalising their world all day, every day. None of us represents a true reflection of reality to ourselves and we have no choice in the matter. Filtering is necessary for survival. Our senses are bombarded by millions of bits of information every second. If we didn't filter out and delete vast amounts of data unconsciously we would be completely overwhelmed.

Every time you filter certain information *in*, you will inadvertently, and automatically filter other information *out*. As a result of your life experience, you will have unconsciously, and accidentally trained yourself to filter for certain things.

When you think of yourself what do you filter for? Good stuff or bad stuff? When you remember your past, what do you filter for? Happy, successful times, or failures and misery?

As a consequence of what you filter in, what gets filtered out? If you filter for all the times your spouse has annoyed you, you will automatically filter out all the times they did things that made you feel great. If you filter for things you hate about yourself, you will automatically filter out things to love about yourself. If you filter for times you felt self-conscious, you will filter out all those times you felt confident. If you filter for the worst in others, you will filter out the best in them. How does the way you filter affect your version of reality, and in turn your behaviour?

Filtering is also a fundamental part of the **structure** of beliefs.

When you have a strongly-held belief, you will automatically filter for all the evidence that supports it, and filter out any contradictory evidence.

If you ask somebody who believes they are highly stressed "when was the last time you felt relaxed?" they will say "never!" This won't be true, but their beliefs about themselves influence their filters.

When somebody has a limiting belief such as "I'm just meant to be overweight", their brain will automatically filter for the evidence that supports that belief, and filter out the evidence that contradicts it.

One of the things you must do when changing limiting beliefs is to filter for the evidence that contradicts them, and supports the beliefs you want to replace them with.

At first this will take effort. If you are in an argument with your spouse and they are filtering for "you don't love me!" and you ask them, "What do I do to prove I love you?" they will shout, "Nothing!"

If you force yourself to start looking for the evidence you will find it, and it will gather momentum. States are linked. When you are in one emotional state it becomes much easier to remember other times you have felt the same way. Once you start filtering for the evidence that supports your new empowering beliefs, it will get easier and easier.

Exercise

» Filter for things you have successfully learnt in the past, especially if they were difficult at first. Write down five examples.

» Filter for the adversity you have overcome in the past. Write down five examples

» Filter for other people who have overcome similar challenges and achieved what you want to achieve. If they can do it, so can you! Write down five examples

» Also, recognise that you can't prove something to be impossible. You can only prove that it hasn't been done *yet*.

The Structure of Beliefs - Imagery

Another key component of the structure of beliefs is imagery – the images, movies, and fantasies that somebody plays out in their mind.

Consider the difference between the following four states:

Hopelessness

To create hopelessness, you play one movie in your mind, and one movie only; you imagine yourself failing and never escaping the rut you are stuck in. You make this movie very big, vivid and detailed so that it feels real.

Doubt

To create doubt you play two movies: one of failure and one of success. But you spend more time playing the failure movie and you make it bigger, brighter, more detailed, more vivid, more real, and you're probably associated (inside your own body in the movie).

Conversely you'll spend less time playing the success movie and you'll make it smaller, duller, perhaps black and white, less detailed, less vivid, less real, and you're probably disassociated (out the movie – as though watching a third person).

Hope

To create hope you also have to play two movies. This time you spend more time on the success movie and you make that one bigger and more powerful than the failure movie.

Positive Certainty

To create positive certainty – when you know 100% that you will succeed, you play one move and one movie only, a success movie. You make this movie big, bright, vivid, detailed and associated.

Reference Experiences

As I mentioned when I spoke about focus and mental rehearsal, if you have been overweight or struggled with your weight for a prolonged period of time, you have lots of experiences in your memory of being overweight. Therefore, when you imagine your future, these images are the freshest in your mind and therefore the easiest for you to create. Remember, if left to its own devices, the mind favours familiarity and the path of least resistance, so it will draw on past experience rather than go through the effort of creating new memories.

You will only change your results when you programme your brain to expect a different outcome. To do this you have to give your brain new reference experiences of you being fit, healthy, athletic and in great shape. You have to experience results in advance.

Once again this brings us back to the importance of mental rehearsal. Spend some time every day imagining yourself having already achieved your goal, as though it were a reality right now. This is a skill you will develop and improve upon.

While you are training yourself in this new way, you may have moments throughout the day where you start to play out those old failure movies in your head again. You must develop greater and greater levels of self-awareness so that you can spot this happening quickly and nip it in the bud. Immediately replace these temporary flashes with positive images and memories from your mental rehearsal sessions. With consistency, this will because easy and automatic.

Rewriting Limiting Beliefs

Here are some typical examples of limiting beliefs:

"I'm meant to be overweight"

"I'm just a shy person"

"My genes make me overweight"

"Fat loss is hard"

"Healthy eating is boring",

"I don't have time"

Many people get hung up arguing about whether their beliefs are true or not, or whether they are right or wrong. This is pointless because the whole point about a belief is that you can't prove whether it is true or not. What you really need to ask yourself is:

"Is it empowering or life enhancing?"

If not, change it.

Write down the new belief. Filter for and write down the evidence that contradicts the old belief and supports the new one. Then direct your imagery and mental rehearsal in a way that supports your new empowering beliefs, the life you want to live and the person you want to become.

Summary

Beliefs are the unconscious filters through which we process information and make decisions. They influence our perception of life, our experience of life, and our ultimate destiny. They control the journey, and the destination.

A person's expectation that they will succeed or fail will affect their physiology as well as their unconscious choices. Beliefs are self-fulfilling.

Many people do not allow themselves to believe in the possibility of success until they have already succeeded. Unfortunately, it is the *belief* that starts the whole process off and dictates the outcome. If you want to succeed you must expect to succeed. You must also *expect* that you will step up and do whatever it takes to find a way to succeed.

Beliefs are simply generalisations. They are not true.

Whenever somebody has a belief or conviction, they will automatically filter for the evidence that supports the belief, and delete or distort any evidence that contradicts that belief.

Beliefs are reinforced by filtering, imagery, and reference experiences. All these can be intentionally manipulated to change our beliefs.

Decide what to believe – about yourself, what you are capable of, and what your future holds. Once you have designed and installed these beliefs, maintain them relentlessly every day by intentionally filtering for supporting evidence, and vividly imagine yourself as already being that way.

Incorporate your new, empowering beliefs into your Unconscious Identity. When you do your mental rehearsal sessions, be sure to incorporate the beliefs you want to reinforce.

4 Stress

What You Will Learn

» Why and how stress puts the brakes on fat loss and body transformation programmes.

» How stress disrupts your hormones and your biochemistry in ways that significantly inhibit fat loss and muscle recovery.

» How stress affects your behaviour and increases the likelihood of self-sabotage.

» How your mindset can dramatically increase or decrease your overall experience of stress.

Stress

Stress is a huge hindrance to your ability to lose body fat. It causes people to gain weight **physiologically** due to the biological changes that occur in your body in response to chronic stress, and **behaviourally,** due to the coping mechanisms that people can develop in an attempt to alleviate stress.

In this chapter we will discuss each of these, and in subsequent chapters we will review some common contributors to stress and what to do about them.

The Biology of Stress and Fat

Your autonomic nervous system manages all the elements of your physiology outside your conscious control. This includes things such as heart rate, the release and balance of hormones, digestion, immune system function and so on.

The autonomic nervous system is further divided into two parts: the Sympathetic Nervous System (SNS) and the Parasympathetic Nervous System (PNS).

The SNS is responsible for high energy, busy, stressful activities. It runs the fight or flight response to stress. The SNS helps to give you energy for a workout, to push through busy periods of work, and the automatic responses to survive a threat or a dangerous situation.

The PNS is responsible for all the calming, healing, and recovering activities including sleep, digestion, and immune system function.

When you activate either the SNS or PNS, you deactivate the other side.

For optimal health, we need an appropriate balance of both. We need to be physically active, exercise, and have the occasional high intensity workout (SNS activity). We also need adequate sleep, as well as periods of recuperation interspersed throughout the day to allow ourselves to recharge mentally, and recover physically (PNS activity).

With our busy lives, many of us are excessively imbalanced on the SNS side, which can lead to problems if the situation is allowed to continue.

As a result of prolonged SNS activity, and consequently PNS suppression, digestion and immune system function also become supressed. Over time this commonly results in digestive problems and/or immune system dysfunction.

The many negative consequences of chronic stress also include increased fat storage, as well as loss of muscle tissue.

Cortisol

Cortisol is an important hormone involved in the stress response and its primary function is to increase blood sugar to give you energy.

However, chronic elevation of cortisol has a number of harmful effects. Firstly, it will encourage the body to prioritise fat storage and fat retention. Secondly it breaks down your muscle tissue.

Muscle tissue is critical to your body transformation. It contributes to your resting metabolism, helps ensure that more of what you eat goes into muscle instead of fat cells, and gives you sexy curves. Loss of muscle tissue on a fat loss plan is a bad sign.

The net result of fat retention or gain, with muscle loss, leads to a flabby, soft, shapeless figure.

Insulin Damage

Insulin is a storage hormone that tells the body to store glucose from your blood in three places – muscle cells, liver cells, or fat cells. For optimal fat loss and muscle recovery, we want the glucose to be stored mostly in muscle or liver cells (insulin sensitivity). When these are full – as in the case of the typical inactive westerner who eats lots of carbohydrate-dense foods – the cells become less responsive to the effects of insulin (insulin resistance), and more of this energy is stored in fat cells instead. If this situation gets pushed further, even the fat cells become more resistant – leaving toxic levels of sugar floating around the blood stream. This is called Type II diabetes.

However, it is still possible for a highly-stressed person to develop insulin resistance on a low carbohydrate diet. Chronic stress can still raise blood sugar levels via the effects of cortisol, and if that sugar is not used for energy throughout the day, the body will release insulin to put it back into storage. Overstimulation of this cycle can cause insulin resistance in the same way as a high carbohydrate intake.

Pregnenolone Steal

Cortisol is created by its mother hormone pregnenolone, which is also used to manufacture the sex hormones testosterone and oestrogen. Unfortunately, as the body has a limited rate of pregnenolone production, during times of stress it will prioritise cortisol over sex hormone production (because evolutionarily, stress meant a life-threatening situation).

This leads to problems with sexual health as well as further exacerbating the issues with fat loss and muscle maintenance or growth.

Stress, Behaviour and Fat

Not only does stress make you fat via physiological mechanisms, it also makes you fat indirectly via mindset and behaviour.

Stress feels unpleasant and unconsciously your mind wants to escape this feeling immediately. It doesn't care about long term consequences it just wants to feel better now. Even if better means "less bad" for a moment.

Many people have learnt to use food as a means of trying to escape, or at least diminish uncomfortable feelings such as boredom, frustration, overwhelm, anxiety, worry, anger, and other stressful emotions.

Not only does food distract them briefly from their problems, it also changes their state biochemically. Their blood sugar changes and consequently their hormones and brain chemistry are affected. Through repetition they have trained their brain to associate food with feeling more comfortable, which ultimately leads to binge eating and emotional eating.

On the other hand, when some people are highly stressed they frequently go for long periods without eating. When they do eat, they often go for high calorie, fat dense and carbohydrate dense foods in large quantities.

If this is an issue for you it *must* be resolved. You must tackle the source of the problem, which means making lasting changes to your mindset and your approach to life.

Causes of Chronic Stress

Not all stress is bad. Our primary concern with regards to fat loss and overall health and wellbeing is *chronic* stress - high stress levels over a long period.

Lack of Sleep

When it comes to increasing fitness, strength, and physical performance, recovery of your nervous system is just as important as muscular recovery. Without sufficient sleep your performance in the gym will stall or regress due to neural fatigue.

Poor sleep is also associated with hormone and related changes that contribute to muscle loss and fat retention or gain: decreased glucose tolerance, decreased insulin sensitivity, increased evening concentrations of cortisol, increased hunger and appetite, and decreased levels of growth hormone.

How much sleep people need varies from person to person, but on average you want to aim for eight hours each night. I appreciate this may not always be achievable for those with long working hours, young children and so on, but the less sleep you get, the more it will affect your results.

Mindset and Chronic Stress

Whilst there are many different causes of chronic stress, the most common and problematic that inhibit long-term fat loss are primarily emotion and lifestyle-related, including overwhelm, perfectionism, and low self-esteem. Later I'll be discussing each of these issues in conjunction with state management and binge eating, as all these topics are interrelated.

Summary

The sympathetic nervous system (SNS) controls the stress response and is responsible for preparing you for a physical response.

The parasympathetic nervous system (PNS) controls healing and recovery and is responsible for sleep, digestion, and the immune system.

Any form of stress, whether physical, chemical, mental or emotional, will trigger a stress response. This activates the SNS and deactivates the PNS. Healing, digestion, and the immune system are supressed, and stress hormones, including adren-aline, nor-adrenaline, and cortisol are released to prepare the body for action.

Chronic, excessively high levels of cortisol will:

» Inhibit fat loss and muscle recovery

» Contribute to insulin resistance, causing further problems with fat loss and muscle recovery

» Disrupt healthy levels of sex hormones, affecting sexual health and further inhibiting fat loss and muscle recovery

Chronic stress often causes people to sabotage their body and health goals. Many people have learnt to use food to manage their stress, and adherence to exercise and the overall programme suffers.

Lack of sleep will inhibit fat loss.

There are many causes of stress, but the ones that consistently cause the most problems in a body transformation programme are mindset-related. This includes issues such as overwhelm, perfectionism, and low self-esteem, all of which are addressed later in this book.

Chapter 5

How The Brain Learns

What You Will Learn

» How you have learnt to sabotage yourself.

» How behaviours that feel out of your control, such as binge eating, are developed.

» You are not flawed or broken.

» How habitual thoughts, feelings, and behaviours that consistently affect your body goals become automatic.

» How those habitual responses can be unlearned and replaced.

How The Brain Learns

Do some of your behaviours feel out of your control? Perhaps binge eating, procrastination, or self-sabotage? If so, are you interested in discovering how to replace these behaviours with others that make you feel good and keep you on track, and make those automatic instead? Understanding how the brain learns, unlearns, and relearns helps you to understand how the techniques in this book work, and how to implement them more effectively.

We all do many things unconsciously. For example, whether you consider yourself to be good at spelling or bad at spelling, do you know *how* you spell? As a quick test, can you verbally recall your telephone number... backwards?

People who are very good at spelling will find this easy. They are good at hallucinating - creating pictures in their mind. More specifically, when they learnt to spell they learnt to create a picture of the word in their mind. People who are bad at spelling typically learnt to spell phonetically - they learnt to spell how the word sounds, so they listen to the syllables and try to work out the letter sequence.

When I was at school we were never taught how to visualise a word. Some kids accidentally stumbled upon spelling visually, it worked, they repeated it, and they got good results. Other kids accidentally stumbled upon spelling phonetically. This produced variable results, but since they didn't know any alternative they stuck with it. Through repetition they became very good at a very poor spelling strategy.

This is a slightly over-simplistic explanation, but you understand my point. You learnt to code the information at the unconscious level - you were not aware of what you were doing. The same applies to a *vast* amount of the rest of our internal world:

> » The way you recall events from the past

> » The information you look for or pay attention to in your day-to-day life

> » Whether you pay more attention to what's happening in the outside world (what you can see, hear and feel in the moment) or the inside world (thinking, imagining, feeling, talking to yourself internally etc)

> » The meanings you associate with certain events

> » The way you automatically react to other people, events and circumstances

> » The way you think about yourself

> » The way you imagine your future

> » and so much more

We all structure our internal world differently, and we do so unconsciously. For example, if you struggle with self-sabotage that feels like it's out of your control, or if you suffer with upsetting feelings that seem to come out of nowhere, it's obviously not your fault. You don't know why or how it's happening - if you did you'd change it. Some people will say "I do know why, it's because of this trauma that I went through", but that doesn't explain how others can suffer the same trauma but come through it and go on to have a completely different experience of life.

The good news is that once you accept you have had some involvement in these results, and you make a full commitment to changing those results (even if that means letting go of your old beliefs), then you have just taken your first step on the road to recovery.

Excellence

To consciously learn a skill, we go through four stages:

1. **Unconscious incompetence**. This basically means that you're rubbish and you don't know it! When you're a toddler you don't know how to drive a car, and you don't know that you don't know how to drive a car

2. **Conscious incompetence**. When you have your first driving lesson, you become brutally aware that you don't know how to drive a car! You become conscious of this fact

3. **Conscious competence**. After a few driving lessons, you are now good at driving a car, but it takes your full concentration. There are a lot of steps and sequences to get right and this requires focus

4. **Unconscious competence**. After you have been driving for long enough you can do it without thinking. You can hold a conversation with your passengers, listen to the radio, and still drive safely and easily. The skill of driving has become unconscious

You progress through the four stages of learning by creating neural pathways, sequences of nerve impulses in your brain and nervous system. A new-born baby has to learn how to walk. Through much trial and error it learns how to activate the correct muscles, in the correct order, to stay upright, balanced and moving forwards. This is an incredibly complicated movement and yet we take it for granted as it has now become entirely unconscious.

As another example, when you are learning how to drive a manual car you have to change gear. A very simplified description of this process would be as follows:

1. Depress the clutch (a process which in itself requires a complicated neural pathway)

2. Find the gear stick without looking for it

3. Move the gear stick into the correct gear

4. Find the biting point of the clutch whilst simultaneously applying the correct amount of revs with the accelerator

5. Gradually release the clutch

This complicated sequence of nerve signals from the brain to the limbs and back to the brain again has to be established. With repetition it becomes organised into a predictable pattern, and with more repetition it becomes stronger and faster. Eventually you do it automatically.

There are many things for which you went through a formal training process like this one, and as such you are conscious of the learning process. There are also many other things that you have learnt without being conscious of the process - such as spelling - that through repetition you become unconsciously competent in (excellent).

Unfortunately, your brain will progress through these stages of learning and build neural pathways for everything you repeat in your life, whether it is useful for you or not.

Binge Eating Strategy

Binge eating and emotional eating are no different. They are a learned response. There are lots of variations on how this can happen, but here is just one example:

» Have insufficient skills in productivity and time management to handle your current workload (productivity is discussed in the chapter on overwhelm)

» Have insufficient awareness and skill in directing and choosing your emotions (state management has a chapter of its own)

» Get given a high workload

» Imagine yourself struggling to complete it, feeling stressed, making mistakes, and missing deadlines. Make this internal movie big, vivid, detailed and scary (mental rehearsal)

» Tell yourself, "I can't do it, it's too much!" (internal dialogue)

» Now you feel stressed and overwhelmed

» Experiment a few times with escaping stress using food. This may be the first time, or you may have developed this part of the strategy years ago

» Learn at an unconscious level that food tempo-rarily makes you feel better, or at least less bad (this is explained in more detail in the binge eating chapter)

» Repeat this process enough times until your unconscious mind learns that food is rapid, reli-able, and effective at diminishing psychological discomfort.

» At this point your brain will store this response as the correct one.

This sequence of thoughts, reactions, and behaviours is a neural pathway. Repeat it enough, and the neural pathway speeds up. Your brain will zip through the above steps until all you are aware of is:

Step 1 – High workload

Step 2 – Insatiable craving, or you may even find your-self eating before you even become consciously aware of what you're doing.

This is why people say things like "I don't know where these feelings came from, they just descended on me!" It's because they have achieved unconscious compe-tence at their problem behaviour. They have achieved excellence!

Unhelpful Excellence

The good news is that if you have problems in your life that seem to be out of your control, such as binge eating, depression, low self-esteem, self-sabotage, anxiety, stress, and so on, there is nothing wrong with you. You are not flawed or broken. You have simply learnt an unhelpful strategy and become excellent at it. Now we need to teach you a new strategy so you become excellent at that one instead.

Neuroplasticity: Rewriting Neural Pathways

Just as neural pathways speed up with repeated use, they also slow down with lack of use, and can even be deleted and replaced if never used again.

For example, let's say you're a keen tennis player, but you are self-taught and learnt some bad habits with your forehand technique. To correct it you have to learn a new technique. You slowly and deliberately rehearse the correct sequence of movements, again and again. This creates a new neural pathway. Each time you repeat this new technique, the new neural pathway gets stronger and faster and the neural pathway connected to the old technique gets slower and weaker. Once you've repeated the new neural pathway enough it becomes fully automatic and completely replaces the old one.

It is also critical to understand that we condition ourselves every day through our behaviour. Elite tennis players still rehearse the basics and practise and reinforce their technique every day. Hitting with good technique is easy for them now, but it is still a skill that they reinforce consistently.

Why Am I Stuck?

Many people become obsessed with *why*. "Why can't I do this? Why do I have this problem? Why do I always do this to myself?"

By now you should understand that the solution does not necessarily lie in the answer to *why*. There are many people out there who understand in intimate detail *why* they have problems, but they still have problems.

The person with the poor tennis forehand doesn't need a more intimate understanding of why they hit a bad forehand. They need a more intimate understanding of *how* to hit a *good* forehand.

The depressed person doesn't need an intimate understanding of *why* they are depressed - that usually makes them more depressed! They need to know *how* to live a happy and fulfilling life.

Understanding *why* can have a use, but only in so far as helping somebody to develop self-awareness, and most importantly, *how* to learn something different.

When I discuss things like overwhelm, perfectionism, binge eating, and low self-esteem, I will answer a few of the *why* questions, but more importantly I will show you *how* to get what you *really* want instead.

However, reading and understanding are not enough. That will give you an intellectual understanding of your problems, but it will not fix your problems. Personal change and breakthroughs are things that must occur in your nervous system. You have to feel it.

Let go of *why* and focus on *how*. Do the exercises throughout this book, and incorporate these skills into your life. Hold yourself to a higher standard and dedicate yourself to acting from the best in you every day. You will be amazed at how quickly you can rewrite neural pathways when you are resolute on doing so.

Summary

There are four stages of learning:

1. Unconscious incompetence
2. Conscious incompetence
3. Conscious competence
4. Unconscious competence

When you achieve unconscious competence, you have achieved excellence – you can produce results automatically without thinking about it.

You will move towards excellence with anything that is repeated over and over whether it is useful and life enhancing, or unhelpful and destructive. This applies to thoughts, emotions, and behaviours. You can be excellent at being overweight, or you can be excellent at being fit and healthy.

Every area in which you produce results automatically is a neural pathway, a sequence of nerve impulses that creates a result, whether useful – as in the case of driving a car, or destructive – as in the case of habitual binge eating.

Neural pathways speed up with repeated use, and slow down with lack of use. This ability for the brain and nervous system to change, update, and evolve is called neuroplasticity.

Neuroplasticity allows us to delete unhelpful neural pathways and replace them with useful ones. Any habitual thought, feeling or behaviour holding you back from the body and the life you want can be changed, regardless of how long it has gone on for, and even if it feels out of your control.

Fully committing yourself to the exercises in this book will allow you to change your neurology in a way that supports your body goals, the person you want to become, and the life you want to live.

Personal change is not an intellectual understanding; it is a neurological event – something that you have to experience and feel inside yourself. That is why reading this book is not enough, you must *action* what you learn.

6 Overwhelm

What You Will Learn

» What causes overwhelm.

» The unconscious processes people engage in that increase feelings of overwhelm.

» How to overcome overwhelm so that you experience less stress, increase your productivity, improve adherence, and accelerate your fat loss results.

Overwhelm

Feeling overwhelmed is one of the most common causes of stress and it is extraordinary how wide-spread it is.

There are, however, people who have great challenges, and great responsibilities, who seem to manage just fine. What is the difference?

Here are just a few elements to the overwhelm strategy. Most people have experienced at least a few of these behaviours:

» You have To Do lists everywhere – pieces of paper with notes scattered everywhere, notes on your phone, on your laptop, some in your head that you remember, others in your head that you can't quite remember and that in itself stresses you out even more

» There is no order to those notes, so you are very reactive to your tasks. Rather than having a clear and efficient strategy you tackle the first thing that comes to mind, or seems the most urgent

» You get repeatedly distracted from your tasks or you suddenly think of another task that seems more important so you drop what you're doing and start that. You have no real progress or sense of completion

» You have no sense of priority so you spend much of your time doing the day-to-day tasks and side-lining the important tasks that will move your life forwards. As such it feels like

Groundhog Day. Plus, because you feel you're just surviving rather than truly chasing life and making real progress towards a better life and a better you, it stresses you out still further

» Since your experience of life so far is that all the stuff you *have to do* stresses you out so much, you want to avoid putting yourself through so much stress. Therefore you procrastinate, hesitate, and your To Do list keeps growing. On top of this now your sense of self, self-esteem, and confidence in your own capabilities is diminished because you accumulate more and more reference experiences of yourself failing to deliver or accomplish your goals

» You waste time and energy on things out of your control, things that haven't even happened yet, or things that happened in the past. Perhaps you worry a lot; you repeatedly imagine what you hope won't happen in the future. Perhaps you feel upset about things that happened in the past by repeatedly remembering those events over and over. So all the time, energy and focus you require for productivity is stolen and wasted through fear, worry, anxiety, and upset. You feel worse, get less done, and feel more stressed

» You chunk things in too much detail. For some people going to the gym is just one task in their head: "After work I'll go to the gym". For others, it is 100 tasks: "Before I go to work I've got to pack my gym stuff, and prepare my post workout shake/meal, then after I finish work I've got to battle my way through rush hour traffic, then I've got to find a parking spot, and it's always busy so I might have to park a few streets away and walk, then I've got to find a free locker, get changed, and do my warm up before I can get started. Once I have started often the kit I want to use is busy so I've got to figure out how I'm going to adjust my programme, then I've got to stretch and do my rehab, then I have to shower, get changed again, battle my way home through traffic again before I even get to start dinner! Maybe I'll skip it this time and order a pizza!" So by chunking tasks in minute detail in your mind you make everything seem much more overwhelming.

I hope you can now appreciate that successful fat loss and body transformation are about so much more than just diet and exercise. You need to grow, develop, and improve as a person and must learning essential life and mindset skills. This is perhaps the biggest cause of failure in the fitness industry: people take their existing mindset, lifestyle, and strategies for how they run themselves and their lives, and try to shoehorn in a diet or training programme.

Your body and your life will not get better until *you* get better.

Overcoming Overwhelm

Broadly speaking, in order to overcome overwhelm and significantly reduce the stress in your life, you need to:

» Improve your **time management**, productivity, and develop efficient systems.

» Improve your **state management**: learn how to direct your feelings and emotions in a useful way, independent of what might be happening around you.

State management is a huge topic and we will discuss it in detail in a later chapter.

Productivity and Time Management

Such a sexy topic, right? Who would have thought that building sexy curves would come down to organisation? However, neglect it at your peril. It's a lot more exciting and stimulating to talk about a brand-new diet, but not only will developing your skills in productivity and time management improve your life, and your experience of life, it will also contribute in a huge way to your body transformation.

Here are some quick tips for making big changes in this area. You may well have heard them before, but as you read each one ask yourself honestly, when was the last time you applied it consistently? In fact, when was the last time you applied every one of these together, every day, for five days in a row?

Get your To Do list in one place. Evernote is excellent for this as it syncs your phone with your laptop. Schedule a review and reorganisation of your To Do list into your diary as a recurring event each week.

Group all of the tasks on your To Do list into areas or headings: Finances, Kids, Household, Social, Fitness,

Career, etc. Chunking like this makes it much easier for your mind to handle, and also helps to ensure you consistently schedule and work on all the areas of your life vision.

Set a clear cut off point between work/productivity time, and recreation/winding down time in the evening. Make sure the last hour before bed helps you to wind down ready for sleep.

At the end of your working/productivity portion of your day, schedule 30 minutes at the end to brain dump and strategise. **Brain dumping** is when you get all outstanding thoughts or tasks, unfinished business, problems, or anything else out of your mind and organised into your notes so you don't spend the rest of the evening running through it all. **Strategising** is when you structure all your tasks and activities for the following day.

Schedule your tasks into focused blocks of work with breaks after each. 50 minutes on, 10 minutes off works well for most people. Do one task at a time and one task only. Do not multitask. During each task switch your phone off, close all social media etc, and be 100% focused and in the moment.

Do not check your emails or messages for the first 60 minutes of the day. These are other people's demands on your time.

Pick no more than two important tasks each day and put these as early in the day as possible, preferably first thing. These are the tasks that really move your life forwards towards your big picture ambitions and goals.

Structure tasks that require less focus, concentration, or creativity later in the day.

Be realistic with the remaining tasks . If you consistently fail to complete your daily tasks you are being unrealistic; this will increase stress and overwhelm, and reduce productivity in the long run.

Decide how you will react emotionally, and what you will do if/when things go wrong. There *will* be days when you get interrupted, or have obstacles and setbacks that chew into your productivity time.

Every time you start a new task, identify the big picture outcomes. E.g. picking the kids up from practice goes from a Have To Do to a Get To Do because you identify the outcomes as; "connect with my kids at a meaningful level, and impart important values to them by asking questions or telling them a story from my life". Also, attach an identity to each task e.g. Supermum or Superdad.

Schedule 10-15 minutes Get Set time at the start of each day. Start by reading through your big picture goals and outcomes for yourself and your life. Get yourself really excited and fiercely driven about where you are headed and your purpose in life. Then review your schedule for the day and make any necessary adjustments.

Schedule the downtime and recovery time I described in the Life Vision section. This is absolutely essential for mental and physical recovery every day. Some people use meditation during this period. Others love to go for a walk, almost as a walking meditation, and either enjoy being in nature, or use the time to listen to an audio book. Walking has the added benefits of increasing your general activity level, as well as helping to change your physical state. If your work keeps you sedentary for most of the day using the walking option is a great idea. The most important thing is that you use this break to recover mentally and switch your brain off completely from anything that feels like work.

Do whatever it takes to get an extra 50 minutes of sleep a night.

This is not always possible for everyone, but it is an ideal to work towards. When you make these behaviours a daily habit, your overall happiness and fulfilment go through the roof. You become more productive - which in turn increases your self-esteem and confidence, gives you more mental clarity and focus, improves your energy, reduces stress and overwhelm and you gain a sense of control and certainty over your life.

Combining Productivity with State Management

If you suffer from stress and overwhelm, you *must* resolve this if you want to lose body fat effectively and completely transform your body. In order to do that you must combine:

» Improved organisation, time management and productivity skills, with

» State management skills – the ability to choose and direct your psychological and emotional state at will, independently of what is happening around you. State management is such a big and important topic that it will have a chapter of its own.

However, understand that productivity and state management are interdependent.

To be productive you must control your psychological and emotional state. You must be able to be completely in the moment and focused exclusively on the task at hand. You must then be able to rapidly switch off and relax when it is time to take a break and recuperate. Then you must be able to rapidly switch mental focus from one task to another so that each task is not inhibited by the one preceding or following it.

At the same time your ability to control your psychological and emotional state is influenced by your productivity and time management. Chaos and disorganisation make it a lot harder to manage your state.

This combination of productivity/time management and state management enables you to handle more, achieve more, and respond to adversity with resilience and resourcefulness, without having to suffer with stress or overwhelm.

All of which makes you leaner!

Summary

Overwhelm is one of the most common causes of stress, and remember that stress inhibits body transformations.

Overwhelm has a strategy. It is not simply a question of how many demands or responsibilities you have. It depends on how you organise both your external and internal worlds.

To overcome overwhelm you must:

» Improve your time management, productivity, and develop more efficient systems. How to do this has been described above. Review this section if necessary.

» Improve your state management: learn how to direct your feelings and emotions in a useful way, independently of what might be happening around you. This is a huge topic and we will discuss it in a chapter of its own.

Binge Eating

What You Will Learn

» What causes binge eating in the first place.

» What reinforces and maintains binge eating.

» Why binge eating feels out of your control.

» What you need to do to overcome binge eating and move beyond it forever.

Binge Eating

Binge eating is one of the biggest obstacles in the body transformation industry.

It is also a dirty little secret for a frightening number of professionals and coaches in the industry too. Many of them have learnt how to get into very impressive shape for a photo shoot or stage show, but only via extreme means. Inevitably this leads to uncontrolled behaviour the rest of the year, binge eating and rebound. When you combine this with a responsibility to be a role model and coach, the impact on self-esteem and integrity can be profoundly harmful.

People typically learn to binge eat in one of two main ways:

» Flawed dieting strategies combined with perfectionism

» Using food as an anaesthetic

Poor Dieting Strategies Combined With Perfectionism

A very common trigger for developing an unhealthy mindset around food is the rules that specific diets impose on people. This is even the case with many seemingly sensible diets and eating plans.

Most diets have rules of some description:

» No carbs

» No fats

» No junk food

» No food after 6pm

» No sugar

Many of these rules, such as zero carb, or excessively low calorie are clearly harmful. If you eliminate an entire macronutrient group you're going to get cravings. If you restrict calories excessively you're going to suffer hunger pangs, cravings, and low energy, in addition to harmful effects on your health and metabolism – all of which lead you to gain more weight in the future.

However, what is less obvious is the harm that even the seemingly more sensible rules create. The benefit of having rigid rules is they eliminate the necessity for thinking and calculation. You don't need an education, you don't need to think for yourself, you just execute the rules and lose weight - easy!

Unfortunately, any time you impose strict rules about how you must eat, you immediately set yourself up for failure because you begin to develop an all or nothing mentality.

You begin to think of foods as being either good or bad. This very easily moves into days being labelled as good and bad days according to whether you follow the rules precisely or not. This can even stretch into labelling yourself as a bad person, weak or lacking in will power if you happen to have a bad day.

This breeds fear of certain foods, and anxiety in many situations where there could be temptation because you always want what you can't have. The longer you keep reminding yourself "don't think about chocolate" the harder it becomes not to think about it!

It is this deprived and restricted mentality created by rigid rules that can easily develop into binge eating. Somebody resists a particular temptation as long as they can, but then when they do give themselves a little slack, all hell breaks loose and they don't seem to be able to stop themselves.

This happens because unconsciously their mind antici-pates another period of restriction and deprivation just around the corner, and it doesn't know when it will be able to get this feeling and this freedom again in the future, so it tries to stockpile as much of that feeling as possible – resulting in a full-on binge.

For some these episodes are not only contained to when they give in to temptation, but also happen when they are taken out of their normal routine and don't have perfect control over what food is available and when, leading to more anxiety, uncertainty and fear.

Early on in somebody's dieting career the initial effects of strict dieting rules are seemingly small and insignificant. When you break them, you simply feel frustrated, but when you repeat that pattern over a few years you start asking yourself "Why can't I do this? What's wrong with me?" That develops into self-doubt, guilt, and anxiety around food.

Add Perfectionism

Some people think the solution is to diet harder, be stricter on themselves, be more disciplined, exert more willpower, and get their diet perfect. The result: perfectionism.

Perfectionism is not the same as having high standards, though many try to convince themselves of that. The biggest mistake the perfectionist makes is that they make the diet the end, instead of a means to an end. They may be aiming to have a lean, fit, healthy body, to feel confident and sexy, to be relaxed around food, and to enjoy life. The perfectionist loses sight of this big picture and makes up their own irrelevant idea of what perfection looks like, and what it means if they don't achieve it. They try desperately to get their diet perfect, and inevitably suffer stress, anxiety, and neurosis. More unconscious feelings of restriction and deprivation, and more binges.

The other thing a perfectionist does is to keep looking for what's wrong with what they're doing: "what else is wrong, what's else could be better?" When you're *doing* perfectionism, nothing ever feels good enough.

For many people, perfectionism is born of insecurity and a fear of being judged: "If I can get everything absolutely perfect then nobody will be able to criticise." This very frequently is combined with an excessive need for control. Some people have trained themselves to need certainty so strongly that they need to feel certain before they try anything. They need guarantees they will not put on weight if they change their diet, that they won't be hurt in love, that their business idea will be a success. They try to control everything in their world to the smallest detail and fear change. The result is stress, anxiety, and the results they are trying so desperately to avoid.

Rigid dieting rules and perfectionism each lead to binge eating and a disordered relationship with food. Combine them and they produce one very unhappy and stressed individual.

What's the Alternative?

Evidently, rules or guidance of some kind are required, or you end up eating whatever you want whenever you want, which is what got you into trouble in the first place. So what's the solution?

Some people in the fitness industry are keen proponents of flexible dieting, or IIFYM (If It Fits Your Macros). You have daily targets for total calories, and totals for your macronutrients (carbs, fats, and protein). As long as your end of day totals meet your targets you have the flexibility to eat what you want.

Scientifically this is a precise and accurate way of doing things. Unfortunately, in practice it neglects the psychological impact it has on most people, and I'm sure you can see the biggest flaw with this approach – it is a massive hassle. You have to weigh, track and measure everything you eat, inputting data into an app all throughout the day. Inevitably, most people either give up, or they eat the same thing every day, which is clearly unsustainable.

Unfortunately, flexible dieting is also another common trigger for perfectionism and a disordered relationship with food, anxiety, and stress. Those people who don't give up or eat the same thing every day can easily become neurotic and obsessive about hitting their number targets and so we are back to our original problem.

The fitness industry has two extreme approaches:

1. A high degree of flexibility, but at the expense of much stricter counting of calories to ensure that you remain within your calorie budget, which inevitably develops into excessive control, neurosis, and perfectionism.

2. Rigid rules that eliminate the necessity for calculations, but which breed a restrictive mindset and train people to think of certain foods or methods as good or bad.

The solution lies between these two extremes. The solution is in fact... drumroll... being sensible, being self-aware, and doing things in moderation! I know! Revolutionary!

Ultimately, we want guidelines, not rules, to help us do the right things most of the time. We want a simple structure - a broad pattern of eating that uses very easy, visual portion control, that incorporates flexibility to substitute foods, as well as to include your favourite treats - in moderation.

The diet of the high performer keeps them on track and within appropriate and easily-achieved boundaries whilst allowing for occasional mistakes, dinners out, wine, chocolate, and all kinds of other delights. Ironically they end up leaner, healthier, and happier.

Once you have established your baseline - a sustainable, broad pattern of eating each week that keeps you on track without suffering with hunger, energy, or cravings - if you need to make adjustments later on you can simply increase or decrease your food intake slightly over the long-term average without having to resort to extremes or knee jerk reactions.

Do not underestimate the results you can achieve with such a seemingly simple approach. At Chase Life we call this approach baseline nutrition, and we have found it to be the most effective way of achieving sustainable, long-term body transformations.

The Anaesthetic

The other reason people develop binge eating is because they have learnt to rely on food as a way of managing their state. Particularly when they feel emotionally stuck.

Firstly, it alters their state biochemically via changes in blood sugar, hormones and neurotransmitters.

Secondly, they learnt that the ritual of eating has an almost hypnotic effect that enables them to zone out and not feel for a while. Food enables them to temporarily diminish or anaesthetise themselves from some kind of emotional discomfort. This could be something as seemingly insignificant as boredom, right through to more intense emotions such as anxiety, fear, worry and anger. Binge eaters often use words such as "not feel", "time to myself", "time to think", and "switch off" when asked what their outcome is in that moment.

Thirdly they may unconsciously have learnt to associate, at a neurological level, the act of eating with a positive state. Many people have learnt to connect comfortable and soothing feelings to food.

People can learn to use food as a means of managing their emotions either by modelling the behaviour of someone else such as a parent, sibling, or role model, or simply through trial and error.

At some point they were faced with a situation where they felt stuck, afraid, overwhelmed, or paralysed by not knowing. They will have experimented with food as a way to get out of emotional pain and move towards comfort. This may not give them the ideal outcome, but as you will discover when we cover internal conflicts later, this was the best choice they were able to perceive, based on that stage in their life and their limited model of the world at that time.

Then through repetition they strengthen and speed up this neural pathway, and food becomes a rapid, reliable, and effective way of changing their emotional state. More often than not, binge eating is less about achieving a positive state, and more about anaesthetising themselves against a negative state because they have not developed any alternative ways of handling adversity or managing their feelings that are as rapid, reliable, or effective.

It is important to understand that the behaviours we are able to perceive as choices are dependent on the state and the context we are in. Therefore, when our binge eater is feeling good and things are going well, they can make choices that support their health goals. But when their back is up against the wall and they are in a pit of emotion, the unconscious part of their mind just wants to feel better *immediately* and suggests the fastest, most reliable way it knows– food.

That is why they must master the ability to manage their state from the inside. Only when they condition themselves to do this powerfully, in the types of situations that used to be an issue for them, and in a way that is at least as *rapid*, *reliable*, and *effective* as food used to be will they change.

Binge eating is effectively a skill. It's a dominant pathway in someone's nervous system. This simply means that more work needs to be done. The great thing about your nervous system is that it is plastic – which means that it is highly mouldable and adaptable.

How Fear Perpetuates Binge Eating

Once somebody has developed the propensity to binge eat, repeating the same strategies and behaviours we've already covered here will obviously reinforce this behaviour, as will mentally rehearsing binge eating – as discussed in an earlier chapter.

However, this is exacerbated still further when dieters are terrified to let go of their current methods for controlling their weight, which have been successful to varying degrees. This is typically the case with the perfectionist who counts calories as precisely as possible, and tries to maintain neurotic levels of control over their diet. In many instances, they have achieved extraordinary success and dramatic transformations. This is very commonly the case with existing and former stage competitors from the world of bikini modelling, and figure competitions, as well as clients of personal trainers who employ the same extreme methods on their clients as they do themselves.

They know that these methods work for them but they are still missing the big picture - that those methods only work for them in the short to medium term, coupled with the fact that they are making them exceedingly miserable!

So they go through periods of being "good" and being "on it" followed by periods of rebound and binge eating. They are so emotionally invested in their old methods that they are terrified of trying something new.

Resolving Binge Eating

Commitment

Training yourself out of these patterns and installing new, life-enhancing responses can be surprisingly rapid when you know how.

To make the absolute commitment required, look at the long-term consequences of your options. If you keep going with the same beliefs, mindset, attitude, strategies (for dieting or managing your emotions), and approaches, what will your life be like in five or ten years' time? Be honest with yourself, as though you were assessing someone else. Ignore what you hope would happen. Forget about meeting someone who could make it all go away for you. Ask yourself honestly; would your life be different if you kept going down the path you are on now?

Then ask yourself; what would happen if you committed 100% to change? What impact will this have on every area of your life, not just your physical body? How will your career, financial life, relationships, social life, recreational life, and intimate life be enhanced and improved?

This ability to be able to assess yourself, your methods, and your results honestly is how you make a genuine commitment, and how you make definitive decisions that change your life. Until you develop that ability to have foresight to the point where you absolutely MUST change, you'll never put in the consistency of effort required to change your behaviours.

Once you are dedicated to a clear, passionate and exciting vision for your life, and make this level of commitment, the rest is just action, feedback and learning.

Physical Hunger vs Emotional Hunger

A key step in resolving binge eating is the ability to differentiate between physical and emotional hunger. Are you hungry because your body genuinely needs fuel and nutrients, or do you want to eat because you want to change your emotional or psychological state? Most people learn the difference simply through self-awareness, but if in doubt, eat a healthy, nutritious meal first (as opposed to a snack – even if you think it's a "healthy" snack). If your cravings disappear your hunger was physical. If you identify it as emotional hunger, there is some mindset work to be done.

What Is Your Outcome?

A client, Miss C, told me of an example of this behaviour when she went to visit a friend in hospital. Her friend was very ill and it was very upsetting to see her that way. Before she knew it, Miss C found herself downstairs in the canteen, buying food out of the vending machine and mindlessly eating.

This is a classic example of using food as an anaesthetic. She was trying to escape the stress and upset. She didn't know what she wanted, and since her mind didn't have a target to aim for, all it could do was try to move away from what she didn't like. Food helped her to "zone out" in the past and so with no other alternative, that's the option she went with.

I asked her what the outcome would be the next time she went to see her friend. Specifically, I wanted her to come up with a clear target for what she wanted to do, and how she wanted to feel.

To begin with she was still stuck in Away From thinking and came up with things like "less overwhelmed", as well as outcomes that were out of her control such as "for my friend to not be ill or in hospital!" Eventually with a little coaching she came up with "I want to be there for my friend, I want to support her, give her strength, and feel love, calmness, and strength".

Now her mind has a clear target. By using the techniques you will learn in the next chapter on state management, she was able to immediately, and powerfully get herself into a state of love, calmness, and strength. We rehearsed this a few times to train this new neural pathway into her nervous system.

The following day she was able to remain with her friend for her entire visit and provide the love and support she needed, without any mindless eating. This skill was not fully automatic or at the level of unconscious competence yet; she had to repeat the techniques several times while she was there to reinforce it. However, she was able to remain completely on track because now she had a much more effective strategy for managing her emotional state and her outcomes, that she was absolutely committed to for her own benefit as well as that of her friend. In a little over two weeks she had completely rewritten these neural pathways and had no more issues with binge eating.

If you identify a craving as emotional hunger, as opposed to physical hunger, ask yourself "what's my outcome?" Very often when someone craves food for emotional reasons it is because they want to diminish, or get away from a negative emotion such as boredom, frustration, overwhelm, or anxiety.

Ask yourself "considering the big picture context of my life, who I want to be and what I want to achieve in the future, what is the most beneficial thing for me to do right now, and how do I want to feel whilst I'm doing it?"

Or "what's my outcome?" for short.

You may identify that you were looking to use food as a way of avoiding the frustration of not knowing how to do a piece of work. Then perhaps you identify what you *really* want is to brainstorm solutions and feel calm, confident, and creative while you find an answer, or find ways of finding an answer.

Or perhaps you decide considering the big picture, I really need to take a break, and to recuperate mentally and physically. Whilst I'm on my break I want to feel a profound sense of peace and relaxation."

Or you may be at a party and ask yourself "what's my outcome?" and answer with "I want to have fun and laugh with my friends, I want to reminisce about old times, find out what's new with them, show them how much I love them, and update them on everything that is new with me". That's a very different outcome to "I'm going to try to resist all the temptation on offer, I really hope I don't break my diet and binge on all that food".

Once you have identified your outcome, you need to commit 100% to the state change you have identified. Which is covered in detail in the next chapter.

Summary

Diets with strict rules and lack of flexibility put the mind into a deprived and restricted state. Inevitably the mind rebels and pushes back, often resulting in a binge.

Thinking of foods as being good or bad perpetuates this cycle.

Perfectionism severely exacerbates binge eating. The perfectionist loses sight of the big picture. The outcome is no longer about achieving a healthy body and mind, and instead all perception of success or failure depends on their ability to achieve their own made up rules of what "perfect" looks like.

Diets that prescribe counting calories (and even macronutrients) are unsustainable long-term and often create similar results in terms of feeling deprived or restricted.

The solution is to learn the art of moderation. People intellectually understand what this means, and often neglect or trivialise it. In practice most people have no idea how to do this.

Binge eating can be learnt as a way of managing your emotional state. Typically, this means using food as a way of reducing or escaping unpleasant feelings. Through repetition this becomes the habitual, dependable method for managing emotion.

Mental rehearsal and fear perpetuate binge eating and create resistance to change.

To resolve binge eating you must:

» Make an absolute commitment to do whatever it takes, no matter how uncomfortable that may seem at times

» Follow a nutritional approach that is simple, flexible, sustainable, and prevents any issues with hunger, energy, or physical cravings

» Learn to differentiate between physical and emotional hunger

» Train yourself in Towards thinking by using the "what's my outcome?" approach

» Master state management, as described in the next chapter

8 State

What You Will Learn

» Why your fat loss and body transformation goals are utterly dependent on your ability to control your mental and emotional state – how you feel from moment to moment.

» What influences how you feel in any given moment.

» How you can learn to switch from a negative or destructive state into a positive, useful, or empowering state immediately, in any situation.

State Management

When I talk about your state, I'm talking about your daily psychological and emotional states.

On the one hand, we have states that are destructive, paralysing, or inhibitory such as boredom, fear, frustration, anger, overwhelm, anxiety, sadness, worry, jealousy, apathy, self-pity, helplessness, hate, or depression.

On the other hand, we have states that are empowering, enabling, and life-enhancing such as joy, passion, humour, enthusiasm, energy, excitement, confidence, inner strength, tenacity, resolve, self-assurance, creativity, curiosity, assertiveness, love, calmness, relaxation, and inner peace.

For most people, their state of mind is something that happens to them. They may attempt to direct their thoughts and feelings to a certain degree but for the most part they are being swept along by the ebb and flow of life, circumstance, the influence of other people, adverts, TV and social media. Something happens and they just respond by going into a state automatically, without any conscious thought to direct their state themselves. For example:

» They have a disagreement with their spouse and find themselves in a state of anger

» They get given a new task at work and find themselves in a state of overwhelm

» They receive their credit card bill and spend the rest of the day in a state of anxiety

» They watch a movie on TV and momentarily get swept along with the story and forget about their life, until the movie finishes and they return to dwelling on their fears and frustrations

» Their spouse wants to be intimate, but they find themselves in a state of self-consciousness or embarrassment and decline, then they find themselves in a state of guilt or frustration

Most of us have learnt that we can create a temporary state change via external means such as eating food, drinking alcohol, smoking, watching TV etc. These methods mostly change our state by changing our biochemistry or distracting us for a moment. But they don't tackle the source of the issue.

When someone is trying to anaesthetise themselves from unpleasant feelings, these could be the more extreme and intense feelings such as depression, but it could also be something as seemingly insignificant as boredom. Both are states that your mind doesn't like and wants to escape (hopefully you spotted the Away From language here).

What would it be like if whenever you find yourself in a state of frustration, overwhelm, sadness, low self-esteem, anxiety, boredom, or stress, you could immediately replace it with confidence, calmness, inner strength, peace, excitement, or passion?

This is absolutely a skill that you can develop; your body transformation goals depend on it (as well as every other goal you have in your life).

State and Weight Loss

So what's the big deal with managing your state? Most people understand some of the more obvious implications, but few people appreciate how far reaching its effects are. Your ability to control your mental and emotional state is critical to your body transformation success for the following reasons:

> » Direct impact on consistency
>
> » Stress
>
> » Indirect impact on consistency
>
> » Resourcefulness

Direct Impact On Consistency

Your state drives your behaviour. The more time you spend in disempowering states, the less control you have over your behaviour. You end up making bad choices that sabotage your body. Here are just a few examples:

> » You feel overwhelmed at work and use food to distract yourself
>
> » You feel bored at home and use food for a bit of stimulation
>
> » You've had a long day and your motivation to train has disappeared and been replaced by a motivation to stay on the couch
>
> » Your spouse is late replying to your messages and you find yourself in a state of jealousy. Your productivity disappears and you seek to comfort yourself with a glass or two of wine

» You suffer with low self-esteem, to the point where you feel extremely upset at times. You use food to console or anaesthetise yourself

» You go out with friends and they apply pressure to get you to drink more or eat more, perhaps by making fun, being upset, or feigning concern. You give in to avoid the humiliation or anxiety

» The kids are misbehaving and you feel stressed so you open a bottle of wine.

» You put weight on after a holiday and feel so upset that you lose faith, and find yourself in a state of doubt or hopelessness. You give your workout a miss because you think "what's the point?"

» Everything has gone wrong and you feel so angry. You should be doing food prep for the next day but you're so angry you think "screw it all!" and don't bother

Stress

As we have explained in detail, chronic stress plays havoc with any body transformation attempt for two reasons:

1. behavioural coping mechanisms, and

2. physiological changes that inhibit fat loss and muscle recovery.

So much of the stress that people experience is because of their mindset. Even people who don't consider themselves to have any major hang ups often create stress without realising it. If on top of this you throw in things like low self-esteem, anxiety, perfectionism, over-analysing, worry and so on, you can begin to understand how people keep piling on the stress. This will significantly improve when someone learns how to better manage their state.

Some people buckle easily under pressure while others can handle high levels of responsibility, work load, and uncertainty, and yet remain calm and in control most of the time. This isn't a genetically-given gift, it is simply how they have learnt to manage their mindset. Some people's lives do indeed have significantly more stressors than others. However, they could reduce the amount of stress their body experiences simply by how they run their brain.

Indirect Impact On Consistency

Sometimes people will think, "all I want is to get skinny and sexy. What does it matter if I'm pissed off with my boss that day?" Here's why:

Some states are neurologically closer to each other than others. When you're frustrated it's quite easy to transition to anger, self-pity, or overwhelm. Equally it's quite easy to transition from humour, to relaxation, or excitement. However, you're much less likely to rapidly transition from a negative state to a positive state without a significant intervention or interruption to that pattern - something that you will learn how to do in this chapter.

This is what I mean by *indirect* impact on consistency: one negative state can easily lead to a chain of emotions that ultimately leads to self-sabotage later in the day. Here are a couple of examples.

You don't like your job, but you're afraid of the insecurity or uncertainty of a career change. You also lack the self-assurance or assertiveness to improve your current job conditions. So, you sacrifice your job satisfaction for job security. There are moments when you're motivated to get lean, fit and healthy, but this motivation is generally suppressed by feelings of unhappiness, lack of fulfilment, lack of purpose, and frustration. So, whilst your fitness seems important at times, at other times it's the last thing you want to think about.

You lack self-esteem and confidence, so you fall into relationships with people who say nice things to you, but who you know aren't good for you. When they treat you poorly you blame them, instead of recognising that if you valued and respected yourself highly enough you would have made very different choices. You then anaesthetise yourself from these upsetting feelings with food and alcohol.

This doesn't mean you have to be like a Buddhist monk 24/7; it's normal and reasonable to be pissed off once in a while. This is not about perfectionism; it is about consistency and results. The better you learn to manage your state and your emotions in all areas, the better your body transformation results.

Resourcefulness

You will have had times when you were in a bad mood, and a particular problem or challenge in your life seemed insurmountable. At another time, when you were in a good mood, that same issue didn't seem so bad. You could handle it, and figured out solutions.

Your resourcefulness depends on your state. In a state of confidence, it is easy to access the resource of creativity - necessary for creating solutions. You will also notice opportunities because confidence puts your mind into a state receptive to possibility. In a state of overwhelm, creativity is neurologically much harder to access. Overwhelm can easily make you blind to possibilities, and lead you into a state of impossibility.

If you want to create a truly fulfilling life that encompasses all your goals, including your body transformation goals, it is vital that you learn to put yourself in resourceful states that consistently support your goals and the life you want to live, and that allow you to act from the best, rather than the worst of you.

Learning to manage your mental and emotional state is the most important skill you can develop in order to succeed in your body transformation goals. I cannot emphasise this enough.

What Is State Control?

My definition of state control is the ability to identify the most beneficial state to be in at any given moment, and to elicit and maintain that state independently of external events or circumstances.

What Influences How You Feel?

There are only two things that influence how you feel in any given moment:

> » Your physiology
> » Your focus

Physiology

Your mental state is influenced by your biochemistry, nerve energy, and posture.

Biochemistry

Two key things that influence your biochemistry are diet and exercise. You will notice that your sense of energy and wellbeing is very different when you manage your blood sugar properly through healthy, quality nutrition and dietary practice. You will also have noticed the natural high you get after a workout as your body is flooded with endorphins, blood flow is increased, deep breathing is increased, and stress hormones are used in a positive way.

Many people have learnt to manipulate their biochemistry and control their state in detrimental ways using things like junk food, alcohol, cigarettes, and even drugs.

Nerve Energy

Just as your muscles need to recover, so does your nervous system. You may have noticed how much more difficult a workout can be after a bad night's sleep.

That's because your nervous system is tired and it is less capable of sending rapid messages to your muscles.

Once again healthy living - good nutrition, adequate sleep and regular exercise - will help.

We can also influence nerve energy with drugs. For instance, many of us regularly consume caffeine, which excites the nervous system.

Biochemistry and nerve energy are very important and we should do what we can to enhance and improve them in healthy ways. However, many people will also use these factors as an excuse as to why their feelings are not their fault:

> "It's not my fault I feel this way, it's my period."

> "Sorry I overreacted but it's not my fault, I'm hungry, I've got low blood sugar."

> "It's not me. I just didn't sleep well."

> "I haven't had my morning coffee yet."

Certain internal and external environments can make managing your state much more challenging. However, we still have a choice. For example, you will have had times when you felt tired or hungry, and all of a sudden there was an emergency, or crisis, or even something exceptionally exciting or captivating, and suddenly you completely forgot about your tiredness or your hunger.

Posture

The key component of your physiology to focus on is your posture. In this context I'm referring to everything you do with your body including how you stand or sit, gestures, facial expression, breathing, voice volume, tonality, and tempo, muscle tension, movement and so on.

Everything you do with your body tells your brain how to feel. We understand that when someone is anxious they have lots of muscle tension, they fidget, and their breathing is rapid and shallow. What we often don't realise is that it works both ways: those physical activities and positions make you feel more anxious.

Here's an exercise to demonstrate this effect.

Exercise

Stand up as tall as you can with your feet shoulder width apart, your arms outstretched as wide as you can to your sides, and your head held high. Breathe slow, deep, full breaths into your abdomen. Notice how this posture makes you feel emotionally. There is no right or wrong answer here; some people feel strong, others confident, others exposed and vulnerable. Once you have identified this, maintain exactly the same posture, but say the opposite to yourself out loud. For example, if this posture makes you feel strong, say "I feel weak" out loud. As you do that, is that true? What you'll find is that simply saying those words doesn't change the reality that you feel strong (in this example) in that posture.

Try it with a very different posture. Sit in a chair, put your elbows on your knees and your head in your hands. Make your breathing shallow and rapid as though you were almost hyperventilating. Once again notice how you feel emotionally in this posture, and then say the opposite out loud starting with "I feel... " Again, notice how even though you say those words, it doesn't change how you feel.

What we learn from this is that what you do with your body tells your brain how to feel and, crucially, it overrides the words that we say to ourselves.

Let's say you are coaching yourself (to be discussed later) and the content of what you are saying is great. You're saying things like, "well done, you are amazing, you can do anything" and so on. However, your posture reflects weakness, low energy and insecurity, and your voice tonality portrays doubt and apathy. Guess which message your brain receives. Your state will remain in weakness, low energy, insecurity, doubt and apathy, since that's the message you are conveying with your physiology.

Your language and your internal dialogue are important, but your physiology *must* convey the state you are committed to feeling.

Now let's say you are using your internal imagery to create calm (also to be discussed later). However, if you keep your body tense, you frown, your breathing is rapid and shallow, you fidget and so on you simply won't experience the state you are trying to create.

You cannot change your state without changing your physiology, and you cannot change your physiology without changing your state. Control of your body is everything.

Let's try some other examples to demonstrate how your body affects your state. Sit or stand in the way that you would if you had extraordinary confidence, energy, and excitement surging through your body. Now sit or stand how you would if you were extraordinarily bored, tired, and consumed with self-doubt. Stay in each posture to make sure you've got it right, and then go back and forth between the two. If you're doing it right and committing to each position, you'll notice a profound difference in how it makes you feel.

Now stand up, take on the most energetic posture you can imagine, and shout "Yes!" at the top of your voice. Don't hold back. Once again if you have committed to this 100% you'll notice a surge of energy in your body and feel the blood tingling in your veins.

Now try this: stand up with the most empowering posture ever. Create a strong base with your feet and legs, keep your torso upright, tall and strong, have your arms relaxed by your sides, bring your shoulders back, lift your head up and look slightly above horizontal with both your head and your eyes, breath in a deep, slow, relaxed manner from your diaphragm, and finally, stick a big, genuine smile on your face - the type of smile that makes your eyes smile. Now you must keep this physiology exactly the same and, as you do so, try to make yourself feel depressed. Notice how difficult this is without changing something about your physiology at the same time.

The fastest way to change your state is to change your physical state, and it is critical that you use everything about your body to create that state. The remaining factors we are about to discuss in this chapter are very important, and yet they are useless if they are not matched with the corresponding posture and physiology.

Congruence is key here. Use every one of the muscles in your body from the small ones that control your facial expression and your voice, to the big ones that control your posture, your movements, your gestures and your breathing to reflect the state you have committed to feeling.

Exercise: Posture and States

See how rapidly and powerfully you can influence your state using your posture. Use your body to cycle through the following three states several times:

1. Calm   2. Confidence   3. Energy

Commit to each state with every cell in your body. Take full advantage of the following variables:

» Body position

» Movements and gestures

» Facial expression and facial tone

» Muscle tension and muscle tone

» Shoulder position

» Breathing rate

If you leave somebody with these instructions and watch them, you'll notice that most people don't even get close to maximising their physical range. What would you look like if you just won the 100m final in the Olympics?

How would you celebrate? Would you shout? Would you pump your fists? Would you jump up and down? *That's* what energy looks like.

When you feel profoundly calm, as you would if you were sitting on a bench, observing beautiful scenery, perhaps a lake, the ocean or a mountain view, how is your physiology? How are you breathing? What is your body position?

When somebody walks into a room, or onto a stage with extraordinary confidence, what do they look like? How do they walk? How do they move? How do they hold themselves? What's their facial expression?

Notice the difference you feel in your state by taking command of your whole posture. Get good at making rapid and profound changes to your state by using your physiology in this way, so that you have it ready whenever you need it.

Focus

The second thing that influences how you feel is what you focus on. We will divide focus into two categories:

> » Filtering
> » Internal representations, which is further divided into internal dialogue and internal movies

Filtering

Filtering will influence what you focus on in the outside world. It will dictate what you notice, and what you fail to notice.

It will also influence what you focus on in the inside world – how you feel about your past as well as how you feel about yourself.

We touched on filtering earlier when we spoke about beliefs, but it's important to have a more thorough understanding of it in the context of your state, and how it in turn affects your weight loss.

Exercise

A great demonstration of the power of filtering is to try the following exercise on a friend. Read the following instructions to them:

"I'd like to do a quick memory test on you.

Close your eyes

In a moment I'll ask you to open your eyes for five seconds. During those five seconds I'd like you to find as many red things in the room as you possibly can. Once those five seconds are up I'd like you to close your eyes and keep your eyes closed while I ask you about all the red things you noticed. Make sense?

OK, open your eyes. 5,4,3,2,1 (count extra slowly so they get perhaps ten seconds, but telling them they were only going to get five puts them under pressure so they scan more quickly and are likely to react more unconsciously).

Now close your eyes and list all the things that you remember that were red.

Keep your eyes closed! Now list off what was *blue*.

What was green?

What was brown?

Open your eyes and look at all the blue, green and brown stuff around you."

What you'll find is that when you are given the instruction to find red things you apply a red filter to your experience.

Red Filter

When you apply your red filter, three things happen:

You find loads of red things, and you notice all sorts of tiny red things that you would never normally have noticed or paid attention to.

Also, because you want to find as many red things as possible, you can sometimes notice things that are almost red but not quite; perhaps they're more orange or pink, but because you're scanning quickly your brain registers them as red.

And finally, because of your red filter, not only does this filter in things that are red, but it also filters out everything else. So things that are blue (or green or brown) don't show up in your internal representation of your experience.

Filtering is a very normal and very important function. Our senses are constantly bombarded by information. Filtering allows us to pay attention to what matters at that moment to the exclusion of everything else.

Nobody represents reality even remotely. We delete, distort, and generalise our experience and we have no choice about it. However, we will use this distorted perception to create a "map of the world" – our version of reality. We will then make decisions based on this version of reality.

One of the biggest mistakes people make is believing that their map of the world is the truth - an accurate representation of reality. For example, the person who is convinced that "everybody thinks my arms are disgusting and is judging me" will filter for all the evidence that supports that belief and filter out any contradictory evidence. This map of the world then becomes reality for them.

Somebody who represents reality in this manner is likely to feel self-conscious, withdraw from social events, lack confidence, miss opportunities, and so on. It could also result in other coping mechanisms to detach themselves from what they consider reality. This could be in the form of a comforting behaviour such as eating, or it could be in the form of a rebellious behaviour such as anger, aggression, defensiveness, or resentment.

Now some people will say to you "oh no I'm a very logical and rational thinker and I only focus on the facts". In which case I would refer you to the work of Daniel Kahneman, whose work on human judgement and cognitive bias won him a share of the 2002 Nobel Prize in economics. The point is that unconscious bias affects everything everyone does. Even the CIA has to constantly check the data they receive from their analysts for unconscious bias, and these are people who have been taught about unconscious bias and trained to minimise it.

The problems occur in our lives when we unconsciously filter in a way that isn't useful or life enhancing. Let's look at a few examples.

Depression

There are many factors that contribute to a state of depression, but filtering is often part of the process.

You sort for bad things, in your past, in your present (as well as imagining them in your future), in yourself, in others and so on. Then we get the same three effects as before:

As with filtering for red things where you find many red things that you'd never normally have noticed, when filtering for bad things you find lots and lots of bad things.

Also, in the same way that orange things can get filtered as red, things that are ambiguous, or could be seen as good or bad will be sorted into the bad box.

And what sorts of things get filtered out? Good things, of course. They are there, they do exist in reality, but just as all the blue, green and brown things got filtered out, so with a "bad things" filter, all the good things don't show up in your version of reality.

If that is how you perceive the world, what decisions will you make? How are you likely to respond in your life? You might stay indoors and shut yourself out from the world, because what's the point of exposing yourself to a world like that? You might be distrustful of other people. You might look for and create fewer opportunities in life, and so on.

Of course, these types of reactions become self-fulfilling; the feedback from your life, and your experience of life is much more likely to be "life sucks" and so the cycle perpetuates itself.

Self-consciousness

Remember when we mentioned that any time you have a strongly-held belief, you will automatically and unconsciously filter for all the evidence that supports that belief, and delete any evidence that contradicts that belief.

Let's say that you have a belief that "everyone always stares at me and makes fun of me behind my back". As a side note it's interesting to recognise that this belief is usually predicated upon a deeper belief that "it's important to care what everybody thinks of me".

Sometimes this belief can even start without an actual real life experience. If you have simply imagined people staring at you and making fun of you lots of times, then as we discussed with mental rehearsal, your brain will think this has actually happened. Someone who glances in your direction might have simply noticed movement and looked up to see who it was. But just as in our sort for red exercise this immediately gets registered as affirmation and reinforcement of your belief that "everyone stares and makes fun of me". If, on the other hand, a stranger comes over and engages in very pleasant conversation with you, your filters will delete this from your representation of reality. I like to call this the fudge factor, where you distort reality so that you can jam it into your existing beliefs.

Now, perhaps another time someone actually does make fun of you. Your reaction? "You see! I told you so! This always happens! People suck!" In fact it's only happened once in the last two years but because you've distorted your representation of reality by filtering for evidence of this belief, filtering out evidence that contradicts that belief, and imagining your belief happening on a frequent basis, your brain thinks it happens all the time.

If that's your version of reality, how are you going to respond to the world? What types of decisions are you likely to make? You'll be very self-conscious. When you walk into a new, unknown environment you'll probably imagine people staring, thereby reinforcing your belief further, but also you're using mental rehearsal to programme shyness, self-consciousness, and anxiety into your behaviour. You'll probably avoid new situations or talking to new people, believing that people are generally nasty and only out for themselves. This will also influence the types of relationships you're likely to have.

Self-belief

I remember catching the summary of a match between Manchester United and Barcelona back when Cristiano Ronaldo was playing for Manchester United. The teams drew 1-1 and when Ronaldo was interviewed after the match he said, "we played much better than they did, we just didn't convert all our chances." When they went back to the studio they pointed out that Ronaldo's perspective of the match was inaccurate. Barcelona had more shots on goal, and more possession.

However, I believe that this is one of the unconscious elements of his strategy that contributes to him being such an exceptional player. No matter what is happening in the game, he is always filtering for the evidence that supports the belief "I'm the best, my team's the best, and we're gonna win!" Which of course makes him play better, play harder, and fight for every inch right to the end of the game.

Choose Life-enhancing Filters

This is a great example of using filtering in a life-enhancing way; happy and successful people have unconsciously learnt to do this automatically. The take-home message about filtering is that we all do it, all the time, every day. None of us represents reality. You have no choice but to filter, delete, distort and generalise your experience. That's how the human brain functions. So if you're going to filter anyway, you might as well train yourself to do it in a way that enhances your life and makes you happier and more successful.

Filtering and Your Body Transformation

What you filter for will directly influence your happiness and enjoyment of life, which indirectly affects your transformation. Unhappy, depressed people generally don't lose weight over the long-term, or make lasting physique transformations.

Secondly, there are filtering behaviours that will directly influence your consistency and compliance with your training, and particularly your diet. For example, a common pattern with people who struggle to lose weight is that they filter for food they can't have. People who find dieting easy will filter for, and focus on what they *can* eat, and filter out everything else. At a restaurant, they may already know they want meat and vegetables so they don't even bother reading the pizza section or the pasta section. They go straight to the steaks. When the dessert menu comes out they don't even look at it, and order a coffee instead. People who struggle to stick to a diet do the exact opposite. They read the dessert menu in detail. They even decide on what they would have if they were allowed to have anything, and they imagine what it would taste like in great detail! That's why they say things like "there's just so much temptation everywhere!" If their friends order a dessert, they look longingly at it, imagining what it must taste like, instead of focusing on the conversation, or something else useful and life-enhancing,.

This kind of filtering is driven by Away From thinking. Consistently training yourself to practise Towards thinking every day is a very important part of changing how you filter.

Here are some other things that people who struggle with their transformation tend to filter for:

» Their failures

» Things that make it hard (or "impossible")

» Things that could go wrong

» Evidence of why they can't do it, or why they're not good enough, or why they're just meant to be fat

Until now, you won't have consciously chosen how you filter your experience, because you've been completely unaware that it's been happening. It's an important process but until now it hasn't had a clear purpose or direction. It's been directed by your upbringing, by your experiences, by your emotions, by your hopes and by your fears.

You will notice that people who have a very clear and very detailed vision for the life they want to live, the person they want to be, and *how* they want to live have more life-enhancing filters and fewer internal conflicts. That's because their unconscious mind has a clear direction.

As you gain more clarity on your life vision, train and condition your mind every day, and become the type of person you want to be, you'll find that many of your unconscious filters will simply rewrite themselves, particularly as you become more self-aware. However, as part of that process you may need to consciously identify and change some of those filters yourself.

Exercise

1. Write down what you have typically filtered for in the past when you think about the following things:

> » Your body

> » Your transformation (e.g. weight loss)

> » Your past

> » Who you are

2. As a consequence, what gets filtered out?

3. If this is the version of reality that you represent to yourself, how will that unconsciously affect the way you interact with the world and other people? What choices and decisions will you make?

4. Now spend some time filtering for life enhancing things in each of these areas and write them down.

5. Now spend a few moments reminding yourself of your Life Vision and how your body goal sits within that life vision. With your mind set on "towards thinking" ask yourself what you can filter for to make yourself even more successful in the pursuit of those goals. What can you filter for in yourself, in others, and in your life?

Note: Remember, when you first start consciously filtering in the opposite direction to what you have done for a long time it may take some effort to begin with. You may automatically respond with "never, nothing, it's useless!" and so on. Stick with it. Remember that states are linked and the more examples you find the easier it will be to find more.

Internal Representations

The second aspect of what you focus on are your internal representations. Information comes in to our five senses from the outside world. It passes through our perceptual filters and we create an internal representation of what happened. In other words, we think!

We experience the outside world through our five senses, and hence the only tools we have available with which to think are an internal representation of these, known as the representational systems. We call these:

» Visual (sight)

» Auditory (sound)

» Kinaesthetic (touch)

» Olfactory (smell)

» Gustatory (taste)

I'm going to simplify the internal representations into Internal Dialogue and Internal Movies, since most of your thoughts take place in one of these – you are either having a conversation with yourself or you are playing images and movies in your mind. For example, when you remember an event, or imagine something happening in the future it usually plays out like a movie in your mind.

Internal Dialogue

Everyone speaks to themselves inside their own head, whether they are conscious of it or not. The question is, does their internal dialogue serve them or not? We often ask our clients, "if you spoke to your friends the way you speak to yourself, would you have any?" Unfortunately, for many people the answer is "most definitely not". So why speak to yourself that way? It serves no purpose and there is no upside.

Even if your internal dialogue is not particularly destructive or problematic, the majority of people's internal dialogue is very underdeveloped.

Types of Internal Dialogue

Questions

Questions are an exceptionally powerful way of directing your focus and your state. Your mind will answer whatever question you ask it. If it doesn't immediately know what the answer is it will come up with potential answers. The trouble is many people ask themselves terrible questions such as:

"Why can't I lose weight?"

"Why can't I do this?"

"Why is this so hard?"

"Why am I such a loser?"

So, their mind answers:

"Maybe it's because you're lazy."

"Maybe it's because you're just meant to be this way."

"Maybe it's because you don't deserve it."

"Maybe it's because you're a pig."

Lousy questions create lousy answers and a lousy state of mind.

It sounds so simple to begin with, but consistently asking useful and empowering questions, and actively searching for the answers is transformational. Here are a few examples:

"How can I get into the best shape of my life and thoroughly enjoy the process?"

153

"Who can I ask / hire / get to help me who will be an excellent coach and support?"

"What's the next step?"

"What skills, attributes, and qualities do I need to develop to achieve what I want?"

"What do I need to do or to find out to make sure I succeed?"

"What do I love about myself?"

"What am I grateful for?"

"What can I learn from this?"

"What are the opportunities in this?"

Asking better questions emphasises the choice and accountability you have for how you feel and the results you get in life, and forces you to filter for what is useful or uplifting, and to look for opportunities and solutions.

When asking empowering questions, it is very important to ask with certainty, expectation of finding an answer, and to ask relentlessly until you figure out the answer.

Coaching

Think of the most valuable coaches you have had in your life - anyone who has taught you something, had your best interests at heart and helped elevate your ability, performance and skill. They could be a parent, teacher, coach, trainer, instructor, or even a friend.

Also, think of some of the most effective and successful coaches you have seen coaching others. What qualities do powerful coaches have? Here are some of the key ones to consider:

» They leave their own problems at the door

» They have your best interests at heart

» They clearly believe in you

» They are completely in the moment and focused on you to the exclusion of all other distractions

» They remind you of the big picture outcomes when necessary

» They keep you focused on what matters most to achieve success

» They are kind, even if high energy and even aggression is appropriate – for instance, a sports coach motivating a team before a match, to make them play their very best

» They are congruent. It's not just what they say it's how they say it. Everything is said with meaning

» They don't take any nonsense or excuses

» They have integrity

» They give valuable feedback instead of criticism

» They use humour and light-heartedness effectively

Think of what a coach says and how they say it: "Yes! You can do this! You can do anything! You are amazing! Let's do this!"

What would it be like if you had the most amazing coach you could ever imagine with you whenever you wanted or needed them? If, any time you were struggling, needed to raise your standards, achieve a higher level, or reassess and re-evaluate, they were there for you, keeping you focused, uplifted and on track?

Well you can have exactly that. You can become your own phenomenal coach. The most elite performers in the world, from athletes to singers to the business elite have coaches to help take them to the next level. However, they do not abdicate their own coaching responsibilities. They understand that they are their most important coach.

You are with yourself 24/7 and whether you recognise it or not you are already coaching yourself. Unfortunately, most people are doing so in a terrible manner. Here are just a few examples of some of the things we discover clients have been saying to themselves on a regular basis:

"You suck"	"Fat bitch!"
"You can't do anything"	"You're so ugly"
"You're useless"	"You're disgusting"
"Just give up"	"You're worthless"
"You'll always be overweight"	"Nobody loves you"
	"You'll always be alone"

What would you do if you had someone on your shoulder saying that sort of thing to you relentlessly? I don't know about you but I'd punch them in the face!

CHAPTER 8 » STATE

Transforming Your Internal Dialogue

If your internal dialogue has been detrimental until now, then training yourself out of this might feel weird, wrong or implausible to begin with. This is normal, and is nothing more than conditioning. You have simply trained yourself to do it this way.

Weird is good. Weird means it's different to what you usually do, and if you've decided that what you usually do isn't working for you then different is great.

Coaching Exercise

Set your countdown timer to 60 seconds. During those 60 seconds, coach yourself out loud in the most amazing, uplifting, and empowering way. Say loads of encouraging things continuously for the full 60 seconds. It doesn't matter if you hesitate, stumble or repeat yourself. What matters is the meaning, intensity, and intention behind what you say. Remember the importance of posture as you do this. Put yourself into the most powerful, uplifting posture imaginable before starting, and maintain that physiology throughout.

The reason I want you to do this out loud is so that you can hear the congruency in your voice. The delivery *must* match the meaning. Your voice quality, volume, tempo, inflection, intensity, and so on, are all part of your physiology. Many people's internal dialogue is so weak and lacks emphasis or meaning, but they are completely unaware of it. You need to learn to do it out loud first before you can internalise it.

Once again don't worry if this feels really strange to begin with. Repeat this exercise a number of times and get the weirdness out of the way early so that you can then focus on the delivery. Whilst you are coaching yourself you must maintain all the qualities of amazing and powerful coaches that we listed above.

Here are a few examples to get you started, but ultimately I want it coming from you:

"Yes!"

"You are amazing!"

"You can do anything!"

"You are so good at..."

"You have such incredible qualities, you are... (list them)"

"You can do whatever you put your mind to!"

"You have everything you need within you!"

"You can do this!"

"Whatever happens, you will find a way!"

"You are warrior!"

"You are a force of nature and the world is a better place with you in it!"

"You were born to make a difference!"

"You have an inner strength that is always there whenever you need it!"

"You are a beautiful, wonderful person!"

"All you need to do is..."

These examples are family friendly, but if swearing adds a level of power, intensity, or congruence that makes it more effective and empowering for you, then use it!

Another excellent way of making this exercise even more powerful is to use music. Find the most uplifting music you can think of and play it full volume to really help you get into your coaching.

Once you are confident you can do this in a powerful way for a full 60 seconds, then start incorporating internal coaching throughout the day whenever it is useful. If in doubt use it anyway and see how much you can elevate your state and your results.

Exercise: Coaching To Change Your State

Any time you notice yourself in a destructive state, coach yourself to change this into the most useful, enhancing state that will produce the best outcome.

As soon as you notice yourself feeling stuck, feeling negative, or struggling with a problem, immediately go through the following steps:

» Detach yourself from the situation, as if you were observing from a third person's perspective. Maintain a big picture perspective - consider your life as a whole in a wider context. If it helps, take a bird's eye view of your life.

» Coach yourself internally, but do so powerfully and congruently as if you were doing the coaching exercise we just did. Commit yourself totally to the coaching role and make sure that your physiology, including your voice (even if it is internal) is congruent. Remember to take on those qualities of powerful coaches. Continue coaching yourself until you create the state you need

» Ask yourself useful and empowering questions. Maintain your detached, big-picture perspective as well as your coaching role as you do this. Identify the useful questions to ask, and then commit to answering or finding out how to answer those questions

I would encourage you to also make use of this exercise even when you don't need it. Using powerful coaching and quality questions as a matter of routine throughout the day is an excellent tool for raising your standards, and achieving greater levels of joy, passion and success in your life.

Internal Movies

When people are recalling events from the past or imagining what might happen in the future, they create an internal experience much like a movie.

How do people manipulate their internal movies, and how does that affect the results they get in life, particularly their weight loss results? A number of things will influence the intensity of your emotion whenever you play an internal movie in your mind, be that a memory from the past, or an imaginary experience. We will discuss four of the key variables here:

» Whether you are associated or disassociated (in or out of the movie)

» The level of detail

» How many times you replay the movie and how many similar movies you play

» How focused or distracted you are when you play the movie

1. Associated or Disassociated (in or out of the movie)

Being associated into a memory or imagined experience means that you are in the movie, looking out through your own eyes, as if you were actually there. Being disassociated means that you are out of the movie, as though watching it from a third person's perspective, or watching yourself on a screen.

Being associated increases the intensity of your feelings and feels more real. When you are disassociated you feel detached. You can increase this detachment by shrinking the image down and moving it further away into the distance.

2. Level of Detail

Remember our five representational systems: visual, auditory, kinaesthetic, olfactory, and gustatory. The more of these you include to build your internal movie, the more real and intense it will feel. The visual, auditory, and kinaesthetic systems tend to have the biggest impact, although olfactory and gustatory are sometimes relevant too. Increasing the level of detail within each representational system will intensify the experience still further.

3. Number of Movies Played

The intensity of emotion produced by a memory or imagined experience is also influenced by how often we replay it, and how many versions and examples we play of similar experiences. Play the same movie or lots of similar movies back to back, over and over, and the intensity increases.

4. Focus

The final factor that influences the intensity of the feelings you get with a memory or fantasy is how focused you are when you play it. If you think about the movie for a brief moment, then get distracted, then return to it, and you continue back and forth in this manner, the intensity of feeling will be less than if you gave it your undivided attention from start to finish.

Memories and Successful Weight Loss

Everybody has memories of success and failure in their past, and other memories that are just neutral. Everybody also has memories that are upsetting and even traumatic, as well as those that are happy and enjoyable.

However, those who ultimately succeed in weight loss learn to filter their past consistently for success, happiness, resourcefulness, and other memories that are uplifting and empowering.

When they remember these events they are associated, add lots of details, play lots of these memories over and over, and are able to focus on them to the exclusion of all other distractions. Applying these four things together to pleasant memories makes the positive feelings associated with them much stronger.

This process achieves four things:

» It reinforces empowering beliefs in their capabilities and in their resourcefulness

» It establishes and reinforces a strong, resilient and capable Unconscious Identity

» It reinforces the behaviours associated with these memories via mental rehearsal

» It puts them into empowering mental and emotional states that support their goals and the life they want to live

Do they remember failures or upsetting events from their past? Sure, they may have moments when they are briefly reminded of them, but most of the time they immediately stop playing those experiences and focus on something more useful instead.

If they do have reason to focus on or recall upsetting events or experiences from the past, they do so in a way that drains all the emotion from the event. They disassociate, and make the image smaller, and further away. They won't play this image any longer than necessary, and whilst they are doing so they will also remind themselves of other, empowering experiences or qualities that they have within themselves.

Replaying the image in this way removes the emotion, allows them to gain a new perspective, and to identify and take away empowering learnings, meanings or beliefs from that experience. As soon as they have learnt something new or decontextualised that event, they immediately switch focus to something else instead.

The Future and Successful Weight Loss

So what do successful people do when they imagine their future?

They imagine successful outcomes. They are associated into the movie each time, making it vivid with lots of details about what they can see, hear and feel. They will play lots of movies of success with different scenarios, different environments, different people, different challenges and obstacles. Every time they will imagine themselves performing excellently and achieving a successful outcome. As they play these movies they will be focused on the movie, to the exclusion of all other distractions, so that it feels even more powerful.

Unsuccessful Weight Loss

It shouldn't take too much imagination to figure out what people who repeatedly fail at weight loss do in relation to both their past and their future.

When they imagine their past they will remind themselves of all their failures, pain, struggle, as well as all kinds of other sad, upsetting, or traumatic events.

As they do so they will be associated into those memories, add lots of detail, play them and lots of other similar experiences lots of times, and give them their full attention and focus.

This is a learned behaviour. Some people have learnt to be more Away From in their thinking. Away From thinking does have its uses, particularly when you consider how humans evolved. If you always kept an eye out for what could go wrong, what could eat you, what could kill you, and so on, you stayed alive long enough to procreate. Unfortunately, some people have over-exercised this muscle, and they need to learn when to switch it off and focus on Towards thinking instead.

By diving into upsetting memories in detail, these people repeatedly get into upsetting states and emotions, with all the disastrous consequences on their body transformation attempts we described at the start of this chapter.

They also focus on everything that could go wrong in the future. They imagine themselves having the same struggles, failing, and repeatedly imagine the worst-case scenario. Not only does this put them into very anxious, helpless, upsetting states, but it also installs failure via mental rehearsal, reinforces limiting beliefs, and diminishes their sense of identity.

Choose Your Movies

Hopefully you can recognise parallels in your own behaviour - not just with regards to your body transformation, but in every area of life, whether we are talking about relationships or your career. Most people have used a combination of the success and the failure strategy, two extremes that sit at either end of a continuum, and it is more a question of which strategy have you practised the most?

The key thing to remember here is that it is *your brain! You* get to choose what you do with it. If you don't like the movies you are playing to yourself, change them! It's very simple to do. It may take a little practice and discipline to begin with, but you'll soon get the hang of it.

Managing Your Focus Throughout The Day

It's extremely important to be able to do this throughout the day, and not just when you think about your body or your fat loss goals.

Things are inevitably going to happen in the course of daily life that trigger flashes of unhelpful images and internal movies that could put you into a negative or destructive state if you allowed yourself to dwell on them. This is normal. Learning to direct your focus and internal movies to what you want and what is useful will mean the difference between feeling self-conscious or feeling confident, feeling anxious or feeling calm, feeling hopeless or feeling determined, feeling overwhelmed or feeling energised and focused.

The first step is self-awareness. Start getting good at spotting when you remember or create upsetting or unhelpful internal movies, stop immediately and direct your focus in a useful way, whether towards a useful memory from the past, something you are looking forward to in the future, or whatever's happening right now - i.e. pay attention to the outside world instead of the inside world.

Exercise: Upgrade your Quality of Life

Step 1

Your quality of life can be measured by the quality of your regular emotions. Take a moment to list them all. Two things are frequently apparent when people do this exercise. Firstly, although they have the capacity for an unlimited range of emotions, their range is very limited. They go to the same emotions every day, on autopilot. Secondly, many people notice they are spending too much time in negative emotions, or certainly emotions that are not enhancing or uplifting their life or their experience of life.

Step 2

Write down a long list of emotions you would like regularly to tap into to enhance the quality of your life, create variety, and raise your overall standards.

Step 3

Set your countdown timer to go off every 30 minutes. Then use your physiology and your focus to create empowering states every time the alarm goes off.

As your ability improves through the day, and throughout the course of the week, see how much more you can intensify these emotions - really go for it 100%. With practice you should be able to dramatically enhance your state in seconds. By making a commitment for just a few seconds every half hour, you can dramatically enhance the quality of every area of your life. In a very short while this will become automatic and become your new standard.

Summary

Your mental and emotional state has a profound impact on your body transformation results. When your emotions are directed by external events, other people and circumstance, your ability to remain consistent is no longer within your control. Your state directs your behaviour. In other words, when you feel crappy you make crappy decisions! Particularly around food and exercise.

Mastering your mental and emotional state is *critical* to your body goals.

My definition of state control is the ability to identify the most beneficial state to be in at any given moment and to elicit and maintain that state independently of external events or circumstances.

There are two things that influence how you feel in any given moment: your physiology, and what you focus on.

The primary mechanisms that we focus on for creating immediate, and powerful state changes are:

» Your posture: commit to your state change with every element of your body including your posture, your movements, your gestures, your facial expression, your muscle tone, your breathing, and your voice

» Your internal dialogue: learn to coach yourself powerfully, and relentlessly until you create the state change you are committed to

» Your internal movies: Immerse yourself in mental imagery that creates the state you want to feel. This could be a time you felt that way in the past, or a whole new experience you create in your mind. Imagine yourself in vivid detail already in the state you want to be in, and act congruently

» Any and every time you find yourself in a negative or destructive state, immediately use your physiology, internal dialogue, and internal movies to create the state change you need.

Self-esteem

What You Will Learn

» Why learning to love yourself comes *first*, and a successful, sustainable body transformation comes *second*.

» What causes and perpetuates low self-esteem.

» How to build and reinforce high self-esteem.

» How to overcome trauma and upsetting events from the past.

» How to totally and completely love and accept yourself, *and* feel excited and motivated about your body transformation goals at the same time.

Low Self-esteem

Low self-esteem is a killer of body transformation programmes. Sticking to a healthy training and nutrition lifestyle will seem pointless to someone who doubts their own self-worth, or fears that they won't be loved, or constantly berates themselves. If they cannot imagine a compelling future for themselves, they won't do much to change it. Their best hope is to attempt to soothe or distract themselves in the short term. Many people will turn to food at this point.

Ultimately at its core, low self-esteem is a state, and just like overwhelm, binge eating, and perfectionism, has a strategy.

Here are some of the typical elements of that strategy using the terminology and topics we have learnt about so far:

Sometimes an event kick-starts the whole process. An extreme (though sadly common) example is abuse. As we discussed earlier the unconscious mind can make generalisations and attach meanings to such events that develop into limiting beliefs: "I'm damaged goods", "This means I'm unlovable", "This means I'll always be overweight", "I'm just a failure" and so on.

At other times, it could be a less severe example such as failing to lose weight. This person has most likely tried several deeply flawed or at best incomplete approaches. However, instead of seeing these events as feedback and information, part of the journey, and a sign to search for more information, they label them as failures, as evidence of their own limitations, and even as having a bearing on their identity. All these generalisations and meanings typically happen unconsciously - outside of their awareness.

> » Once they have these limiting beliefs they automatically filter for all the evidence that supports them

> » When they remember their past they filter for their failures, mistakes, and upsetting events

> » When they think of their own appearance, attributes, qualities, or personality traits, they filter for all the things they don't like

> » When they imagine their future, they imagine themselves and their life staying the same or even getting worse

> » Their internal dialogue is terrible; they say nasty things to themselves over and over again

> » Their posture is self-deprecating, weak, submissive, and lacks energy, power or strength

It's all a very convincing story they have been telling themselves which, through years of repetition, they have mistaken for the truth. This story does not define your life. *You* define your life. *You* decide.

So what's the solution? I will summarise the key steps from what we have covered so far, before taking you through some additional experiences that can help speed your inner transformation (which in turn will enable your physical transformation).

Beliefs

Identify the limiting beliefs you have built up about yourself. Recognise that these are not facts, they are not true, they are not correct. They are generalisations that were installed incorrectly and accidentally. If they are not useful, change them! Go through the belief-changing process.

State

Identify the antidote state(s). What state or group of states would you like to experience more of that would transform your life and your relationship with yourself? Confidence is often a key one. What else? Inner strength, joy, humour, love, tenacity? Use the skills and techniques you learnt in state control to create these states within yourself. Do this throughout the day, practising making those states stronger and stronger.

Rapidly spot any time you use your internal dialogue, posture, or internal movies in a destructive way, and immediately intervene with your antidote states - every single time.

Mental Rehearsal

Use the mental rehearsal exercise to install a new Unconscious Identity and a compelling, exciting future. Do this frequently enough that it dominates and over-whelms any old references, and becomes your new default reference point.

More Ways to Build and Reinforce High Self-esteem

Take Action!

This is not an optional extra. It is a necessity. Once you have begun the work to rebuild your own sense of self-esteem, self-worth, and self-love, you *must* back it up with action. You cannot sit back and wait for life to happen to you.

Believing you deserve the best but doing nothing to back up that sense of worthiness is a false sense of entitlement. Ultimately it will implode on itself and result in low self-esteem again.

When you take ownership of your results, you gather more and more reference experiences that reinforce the belief that "I am amazing and I can do anything!"

When you fail to take action in alignment with your new sense of identity and self-belief, it breaks your promises to yourself over and over again. It chips away at your integrity and you gather reference experiences that contradict that sense of self-worth.

Love yourself and believe in yourself, but make sure your actions back it up. Once you have created your strong sense of identity, ask yourself, how would a person who thinks and feels that way about themselves act?

» They do the right thing by themselves, even if that risks upsetting people

» They have the ability to say "no" when necessary

» They stand up for themselves

» They face their fears head on and take action that they know in their heart is right, is in alignment with their values, their goals, and the life they want to live. This could mean talking to a stranger, striking up a new relationship, exiting a destructive relationship, starting a business, or asking for a pay rise

» They love and take care of others, but they love and take care of themselves first

» There is only a small number of people whose opinions they *consider*. Those opinions are *considered* - they are not taken as absolute. They make their own decisions

» They lead their life. They do not wait for a better one to fall into their lap. They go out and make it happen.

» They take ownership of their results, but they are also kind to themselves. They give themselves permission to make mistakes, and they fully believe there is no such thing as failure, only feedback and information.

Make your own additions to this list and read them every day. Make a commitment to yourself to act in accordance with this identity every day. Don't get it perfect - that's impossible – but get it done. Learn, grow, make mistakes, learn some more, and enjoy the process of building yourself intentionally every day.

I Love You

People with severe low self-esteem have great difficulty saying "I love you" to themselves to begin with. It feels so weird, and even wrong. This initial resistance is nothing more than conditioning. They've been so used to saying nasty things to themselves that when they first say "I love you" they don't trust it.

It's not surprising really. If you had someone on your shoulder 24/7 saying "you suck, you're disgusting, you're worthless" and then one day they turned around and said "I love you" of course you wouldn't believe them!

This exercise will feel very strange to begin with. I want you to write a letter to yourself apologising for how you have treated yourself. Explain that none of it was true, that you were scared and hurting and lashed out. Explain that you truly love yourself, write down all the reasons why and say that you know in your heart that you are worthy of love.

Next I want you to stand in front of the mirror and read the letter to yourself - looking yourself in the eyes as you do. Say it with meaning. This is training, so if it doesn't sound right, simply do it again and make the necessary changes to your posture, voice and facial expression so that the congruence is there.

Now put your letter down and stand facing the mirror. Close your eyes and picture someone standing in front of you whom you love with all your heart. Say "I love you" to that person out loud three times. The first time pay attention to your voice. The second time pay attention to your body - your posture, breathing rate, and facial expression. The third time pay attention to where you feel the love in your body. Look into your eyes in the mirror, and say "I love you" to yourself out loud three times. The first time make sure your voice exactly matches how you said it before. The second time make sure your body matches. The third time pay attention to feeling that love in the same location and with the same qualities in your body. Continue alternating back and forth between saying "I love you" to this person with your eyes closed, and then "I love you" to yourself until you really start to feel the congruence and meaning coming through.

Filtering For Self-love

You may have heard of keeping a gratitude journal where you write down things you are grateful for every day. Well, I would like you to do a similar exercise for self-love, only we are going to add another dimension to make it more powerful, because simply making a list isn't enough on its own.

I would like you to start the journal today by writing at least 10 things you love about yourself. Include everything - things about your appearance, your qualities, attributes, abilities, and internal resources.

An additional step which can really help is to close your eyes and picture someone in front of you whom you know loves you with all their heart. Imagine floating out of your body and into theirs. See yourself through their eyes. See yourself through the eyes of love, and then add more to your list from their perspective.

Feel free to also ask family and friends for suggestions.

Each morning choose three examples of things you love about yourself from your list. Imagine you are experiencing each one in turn. Absorb yourself into what you can see, hear, and feel, and allow the physical sensations triggered by this process to flow throughout your body. Continue focusing on each one in turn, allowing the physical sensations to increase each time. Amplify those feelings until you have a full-body experience.

Now imagine yourself moving into your day with that feeling permeating your entire being. How would it change your experience of the day? What would you do differently? What would be better?

In addition, I would like you to continue adding to your self-love journal every day as you continue to think of more and more things to love about yourself.

Overcoming The Past

There can be events from the past that continue to affect your self-esteem today. This could be upsetting and traumatic events that happened to you, things you labelled as mistakes or failures, things you regret, or things you feel guilty about.

The more you focus on upsetting things, the more upset you become. Remember when we discussed internal movies and gave the examples of two people on a body transformation programme. The person who got terrible results filtered for and focused on all their failures from the past, and that's why they suffered and struggled so much.

If you take an upsetting event from the past, associate into it, add lots of details, and replay it over and over, as far as your nervous system is concerned that's reliving it over and over again.

Occasionally there is value in revisiting an event *in a different way*, to facilitate taking new learnings and meanings from it to change old beliefs and build new ones, and to change key decisions that were made at that time. However, in the vast majority of cases, the problem persists simply because you keep torturing yourself with upsetting movies! You are using mental rehearsal to programme misery!

Stop replaying those events immediately, and replace them with what you do want instead - as we discussed in state control. Do this consistently, and with time those old events will fade into the background to the point where they feel like a distant memory, almost like it was a different lifetime or even as though it were someone else.

However, on occasion these memories can become anchored to things that happen regularly in your daily life, and you keep getting reminded of them. You can still resolve this in the same way but it makes for a lot of work. To help drain the emotion out of these memories, and make it easier to let them go, we can use the following process:

Exercise: Overcoming The Past

Step 1
Access resourceful states

Identify the antidote states that would allow you to remember that memory without being negatively affected. Confidence, calmness, and inner strength are often useful. If it is appropriate humour can be an extremely powerful addition.

Close your eyes and take yourself back to a time when you felt each of those resource states in turn. Recreate each moment vividly, adding lots of details to what you can see, hear and feel. As you do so adopt a supremely empowering posture, facial expression and breathing pattern that is in alignment with those states.

Step 2
Disassociate

Close your eyes and imagine yourself in a cinema. Sit down half way back from the screen. If we are working on a particularly strong or upsetting event, sit at the back of the cinema and push the cinema screen further away so that it is a lot smaller.

Step 3
Play the movie on fast forward, disassociated, and black and white

In this step you will play a movie on the screen of yourself in the upsetting event that you wish to work on. Before you do so, mark two points on the movie: one before the event where you knew you were safe and well, and one after the event where again, you knew you were safe and well. These will be your start and finish points. When you play the movie make the movie black and white and a bit grainy.

Before you start, and throughout this whole process, put yourself into your super-empowered physiology to enable you to feel completely different as you watch it.

When you are ready to start, make sure you remain disassociated, with that you on the screen way off in the distance, and that you emphasise playing it on fast forward extremely quickly. Finish at your end point where you are safe and well.

Step 4
Rewind the movie quickly

Rewind the above movie back to your start point again. Once again emphasise doing this extremely quickly, disassociated. Make sure the entire thing happens backwards. Things fall upwards, people walk backwards very fast, the sounds are funny and backwards and so on.

Step 5
Repeat Steps 3 and 4 at least 12 times

Continue fast forwarding and rewinding this movie back and forth, getting faster and faster, and more and more ridiculous with each one. If there is a particular person who upset you, dress them up like a pink unicorn or something else utterly ridiculous. Add silly or uplifting music that makes you smile.

The key with this process is to emphasise the speed of fast forward and rewind, and the level of humour or ridiculousness. Remember to also maintain your empow-ering posture and physiology throughout.

Part of the reason you were stuck with the same feel-ings for the old memory is that you kept replaying it in the same way - associated, detailed, etc. By repeating that process, you trained your nervous system to react the same way to it over and over again. By scrambling the pattern in the way we just have, you completely scramble the old neural pathway which prevents your mind from being able to re-access the information in the same way it used to.

Optional Exit

At this point it should be a lot easier to manage your state going forwards. If you do become reminded of the event again it should feel very different, and you should be able to apply your state management techniques much more quickly and easily.

If the event was one that you had perhaps labelled as a mistake or failure where you had some control or involve-ment in the outcome that, if changed, would create a completely different outcome, then you can move on to Step 6 onwards to install a new behaviour or response in similar situations in the future:

Step 6
Sit down in the front row of the cinema with a completely clean, blank screen and create an image of the new you on the screen

Put yourself into your supremely empowering posture, and as you do so, pour those strong, confident, empowering feelings into that you on the screen. Make that you look and sound exactly the way that you want to see and hear yourself. Notice how your posture has changed, how you move and hold yourself differently, how you sound different, and so on.

Step 7
Play a completely new movie of yourself in a similar situation, only this time behaving exactly the way you want

Make that you on the screen behave and react in exactly the way that you would like to see and hear yourself. Repeat this process until you get it exactly the way you want it.

Step 8
Associate into that movie

Replay exactly the same movie only this time whilst associated so that you can feel what it feels like to think, feel, and respond in this whole new way. Once again repeat this process until it is exactly the way you want it to feel.

Unhappiness and Motivation

Poor body image is commonplace and not useful or necessary. Occasionally somebody says "but if I learn to appreciate myself as I am then I won't be motivated to change". So, we need to differentiate between poor body image and Push motivation.

Now let's be honest - this is a book about transforming your body, and for most people this is about their appearance first and foremost. So there is a presupposition that how you look is important to you. Is that a bad thing? It depends on the impact it has in your life, and whether you set the game up to win or lose.

The person with a poor body image has simply trained themselves to focus repeatedly on what they don't like. Just like the perfectionist, they constantly ask themselves "what's wrong? what's not good enough?" They find lots of things to hate about themselves, with even small inconsequential things coming sharply into focus. As a result, all the things they could learn to love and appreciate in themselves are deleted, or become utterly unappreciated. This becomes a dominant pattern that persists, and even if they succeed in transforming their body, they remain unhappy, ungrateful, and unsatisfied. This can often leak out into other behaviours such as insecurity, jealousy, or self-consciousness and shyness.

Once again this is simply a strategy. They have distorted their reality in a way that makes them suffer unnecessarily. Nick Vujicic was born with no arms and no legs. Unsurprisingly he went through some very dark times in his life. He is now a motivational speaker and lives an extraordinary, and happy life. Look him up on YouTube for some incredible motivation.

Now, imagine for a moment that you had an accident that made you lose your limbs. How would that feel? I bet you would be longing to be returned to how you are right now. You would suddenly appreciate everything you previously took for granted. And yet Nick is happy. Why? Because he directs laser focus into what he is grateful for, what he can do, and on his purpose.

This is an extreme example to illustrate a point. Lots of people will say to you "there's always somebody worse off than you" but for somebody with poor body image, that doesn't make them feel any better or change their life does it? That's because they've trained themselves to focus on what they hate about themselves and until they believe they can change this behaviour, see the value in doing so, and commit themselves to doing so, nothing will change.

Now, some people mistakenly believe that poor body image and hating yourself is necessary in order to be motivated to change. It absolutely is not! Effective Push motivation is about consequences of behaviour, not who you are, or your identity. It is supposed to be empowering, not disempowering.

Push motivation is powerful and important. It usually kick-starts us into action. However, it can diminish over time because as we make progress our everyday experience of our Push motivation is reduced. You can sustain Push motivation over the long-term by transporting yourself into the future and briefly - in the specific moments when it matters - imagine the consequences if you didn't remain on track.

Of course if we spend all our time imagining this worst-case scenario, we're just using mental rehearsal to programme failure. So it is important that this is vivid and powerful, but also that we only use it when it matters. Techniques such as repatterning will help to attach these images to the triggers that used to sabotage us in the past, but the rest of the time we can focus on our Pull motivation.

Use your Push motivation to kick start you into action, then focus your attention on the action itself, what you are moving towards, and feeling empowered. Continuing to berate yourself after you've committed to your course of action is pointless.

Both Push and Pull motivation are important and relevant to everyone. However, some people rely predominantly on Push motivation. For example, they may think, "I hate being overweight, and I hate dieting, which one do I hate the least? I'll do that one." In this example the person is caught in a bind and choosing between the lesser of two evils. Whichever choice they make, the presupposition is that they will still suffer.

Other people rely more strongly on Pull motivation. This might be someone who thinks "I love myself and I am very comfortable in my own skin, but I am particularly excited about making this next improvement".

Obviously, we all have both extremes within us, but when you spend most of your time focusing on what you don't like, you spend most of your time feeling pretty crappy. People who are motivated in this manner tend to be unhappier. Occasionally they get results through sheer force of will, but in our experience they are more likely to sabotage themselves, purely because they spend more time in upsetting states, which can easily spiral into further negative states and all the coping mechanisms we discussed before.

Is it appropriate to have moments of dissatisfaction with your current condition? Absolutely - that can be a useful source of Push motivation. Is it useful for somebody who is so overweight they have made themselves diabetic to think "what they hell have I done? I vow never to do this to myself ever again. I'll do whatever it takes to turn myself, my health and my life around"? Of course it is. But it is only useful if it is used in an empowering way, and if it meets the following criteria:

» It is something within your control (e.g. being overweight as opposed to being short)

» You use the emotion in an empowering way. You don't dwell on it and go into a pit of despair – you briefly focus on it, feel the motivation, make a definitive decision, and then execute your plan

» You don't allow it to define you as a person

You will be much more effective at transforming your body as well as your overall sense of happiness and fulfilment when you start from a place of gratitude and self-love, and focus on building the life you want and being the person you want to be.

Learn to love and appreciate yourself, and be grateful for all the amazing qualities you have. If you are over-weight or out of shape, recognise that that is a reflection of how you lived your life in the past. It does not define you, your life, or your future. You get to decide what defines you and you get to design your future in exactly the way you want it to be. You can totally and completely love and accept yourself, *and* be motivated and excited about transforming your body into a lean, healthy, fit you, *and* enjoy the process.

Summary

Low self-esteem is simply a belief or collection of beliefs about who you are, what you are capable of, or what your own perceived value is. As convincing as it felt, low self-esteem is nothing more than a story you repeatedly told yourself until you mistook it for reality.

To build high self-esteem:

» Identify the limiting beliefs and commit to the belief-changing processes described in this book

» Dedicate yourself to mastering your state, not just when it is convenient or easy to do so, but relentlessly and consistently

» Practise mental rehearsal every day to build a phenomenal Unconscious Identity filled with confidence, self-love, worthiness, inner strength, and empowerment

» Take action! Back up your new sense of identity, self-love and worthiness with congruent action. Mentally refer to your Unconscious Identity throughout the day and consciously act in accordance with it

» Do the *I love you* exercise

» Do the *self-love* exercise

» If your self-esteem is affected by an upsetting event from the past, use the *overcoming the past* exercise to change the way your brain represents and remembers that event

Low self-esteem, self-hate, or poor body image are *not* effective motivators. You do NOT need to hate yourself in order to be motivated to transform your body. You can absolutely learn to love yourself, feel immense gratitude for what you have and where you are in life, at the same time as feeling excited and highly motivated about making changes in the future. This is a much more successful strategy.

10 | Purpose

What You Will Learn

» Why a life of meaning and purpose is important in sustainable body transformations.

» How to discover your purpose.

Purpose

We all know by now that chronic stress is one of the biggest contributors to obesity and resistance to fat loss – through behavioural or physiological mechanisms, or both. For many people this stress arises because they have no clear sense of purpose. They get caught up in the day to day – paying the bills, keeping the boss happy, keeping the children quiet and so on. If they have any time left over it is often spent in a state of exhaustion or recovery.

There is a difference between surviving and living. When someone lacks meaning, purpose, or a clear mission in life, they end up getting caught up in surviving. They chase the endless tasks on the To Do list and often accumulate responsibilities without any clear idea why, other than somebody else expects them to, or they feel they should.

They lose track of who they are and their true purpose. This frequently leads to coping mechanisms used for distraction, such as taking on or creating excessive workloads, emotional eating, or alcohol abuse.

A purpose is necessary for people to wake up every morning feeling energised, motivated, and focused. It gives you meaning, value and creates a life of passion, direction and energy. All decisions and priorities are measured against your purpose and your values. Life becomes simpler, easier, and you experience less internal conflict. You establish one of the fundamental ingredients of *happiness!* Stress diminishes and transforming your body becomes so much easier as a consequence.

You Decide

Whether you believe that your purpose is something given to you by a force greater than you, or whether you believe you are in control of your own destiny, your purpose is something you decide.

If you believe in fate, or a higher power, you still have a choice to make, but you are fated to make the choices that are in alignment with your destiny. You would only make the choices that feel right.

If you do not believe in those things and believe that you make your own destiny, then... you decide!

In either case, your purpose is a choice. It is something you must decide for yourself and focus on the fulfilment of that purpose.

However, because it is a choice, you get to change your mind if you wish! Your purpose is not set in stone, and you can have a different purpose or mission for different chapters of your life.

Some people get stressed and anxious because they don't know what their passion is, what they are here to do. They are waiting for the answer to fall into their lap or for someone to tell them. If you don't know what your purpose is then you either have not had enough experience, or you have not had the right type of experience.

Get Curious, Learn, and Experiment

Whatever your age, it is totally OK not to know what your purpose is yet. Get curious. This is an exciting time! You get to choose your destiny. You get to design your life. So get out there and discover new things, learn, and experiment. Find out what you like, what interests you, and what excites you. This is an information-gathering stage before you take action. Whilst you are gathering information do not concern yourself with forcing a decision. Be OK with not knowing and relax.

Often you don't know how passionate you can be about something until you learn enough about it. I have a friend who is a TV presenter, who was never interested in mixed martial arts (MMA). She thought it was just a couple of guys weirdly rolling around on the floor.

Then she got offered a job to present an MMA magazine show on TV. She had six weeks to learn as much as she could about the sport and the fighters. Being a consummate professional she threw herself into her research and before long she completely fell in love with the sport. Once she understood enough about it she became completely engrossed. She now lives and breathes MMA, is heavily involved both professionally and personally, and has become a well-respected authority.

While you are in this information gathering stage, investigate, experiment, and learn about things that intrigue you. See if that spark of intrigue develops into a flame.

Take Action

Many people get stuck in the information-gathering stage and over-analyse everything. To be honest, in most cases they're not even gathering information or trying things, they are stuck at home worrying and second guessing themselves instead of getting out there in the real world and having real experiences.

You will have much more success in finding what you really enjoy, and what gives your life meaning by throwing yourself completely into things for a period of time.

It is never wasted experience. Firstly, you will develop a variety of useful skills that will remain with you and that you can transfer to other areas of your life.

Secondly, you will be much more motivated and have a heightened sense of integrity and self-worth. When you do something to the best of your ability you get to feel really good about yourself. You are more engaged in the activity, and motivation increases. You also get much better results, and you learn much faster. As your skill, knowledge, and ability increase in this area you typically enjoy it more - we tend to enjoy things we are good at.

Thirdly, you learn if it is really something that you are passionate about and whether it can become your purpose. If it is, great! Continue on your path and get better!

If not, you will have had some valuable insights that will help in your next choice. Plus, you will have developed a whole bunch of new life skills, as well as confidence in yourself, your ability to commit, and your ability to get results and make things happen.

So don't procrastinate on choosing your path. Once you have done an appropriate amount of information-gathering, pick something, take bold action, make mistakes, and find out through committed trial and error. Remember, YOU get to decide what your purpose is. Don't wait for it to come to you. Get out there and discover it.

I am a big fan of the original Facebook mantra: "Move fast and break things!"

What better way to counteract procrastination and perfectionism?

Begin to Decide

What is your purpose? To be an extraordinary mother or father? To discover the secret lives and the migration patterns of whale sharks? To revolutionise the banking industry? To transform 1,000 lives through health and fitness? To entertain and inspire children through children's books and stories? To bring joy and laughter through stand-up comedy?

Your purpose can be multifaceted and different for different periods of your life. For example, it is very common for women to have "being a mother" as their primary purpose. Which is wonderful, but if that is your only purpose it can also leave a void when the children leave home. You will always be a parent, but as your time frees up, we want your life to be filled with things that continue to give meaning and purpose, instead of just keeping you busy.

This doesn't have to be huge or something that others would collectively consider to be profound. What is most important is that your purpose is founded in what makes *you* feel passionate. Be honest to yourself, what you truly value, and what gets you going.

Get out a sheet of paper and write down the following:

"My purpose and mission in life is... "

If you don't completely know what the answer is, go into brainstorming mode and write down as many versions as you can think of. Don't overthink, just write as rapidly as you can.

Review your purpose and mission statement every day, even if only briefly, until you come up with a description that feels right. Continue refining it until you arrive at a sentence that speaks to both your head and your heart.

Once you have your mission statement, put it somewhere prominent and commit to reading it every day. You will unconsciously organise and fine-tune your experience and harness the power of your internal compass - called the reticular activating system. This is a part of your mind that tells you what's important, what to pay attention to and focus on, and where to direct your energy.

Update and Evolve Your Purpose

As you develop and grow as a person, it is only natural that your purpose and mission in life will also develop and grow. You can, and should, review and update your purpose and mission statement as you learn more about yourself, the world, and what you *really* want.

Summary

Without purpose people often create stressful lives, or slip into destructive states such as anxiety, low self-esteem, and even depression because their life lacks meaning and direction. This frequently leads to coping mechanisms for escaping that stress such as taking on or creating excessive workloads in order to keep busy, or binge eating, emotional eating, or excessive alcohol consumption.

Your purpose will not fall into your lap. You decide what your purpose is. You must get out there, live life, expand your comfort zone, explore, experiment, play, and discover.

Do not be in a rush to identify your purpose. Most people venture down multiple paths before they discover their life's mission.

Whichever path you decide on in the short term, commit yourself 100%. Do not do things by half. Live a life of passion. You will achieve more and find out more about yourself, all of which will help you discover your true purpose more quickly in the future.

Your purpose can change as you go through different stages in life.

Update and evolve your purpose and your personal mission statement as you gain new experience and learn more about yourself and what you *really* want.

Chapter 1

Obstacles and Setbacks

What You Will Learn

» Why obstacles and setbacks are inevitable.

» How to overcome them, prevent them from sabotaging your ultimate success, and how to use them to make you *more* successful.

» How to preempt foreseeable obstacles and setbacks and prepare yourself in advance.

Obstacles and Setbacks

It doesn't matter what your goal is, if it's big enough and important enough, you are going to get some obstacles and setbacks. That's just part of the journey. You have to earn your results by your ability to be diligent, persistent, and tenacious. How you respond to, react to and overcome obstacles and setbacks is a critical skill that needs to be developed and reinforced in the right way if you are to transform your body for the long term.

Firstly, you must develop and maintain the skills, techniques, and habits we have already covered in this book including:

State

If every time something goes wrong or unexpectedly you get upset, angry, sad, defeated, or deflated, and then as a consequence give up, procrastinate, or sabotage yourself in some way, then clearly you have some state management issues! It is normal and inevitable for you to feel some kind of a negative emotion such as these when things go wrong. But if you stay there, and allow that to lead to poor decisions, a victim mentality, helplessness, or capitulation then you have some personal growth to do. The moment you notice a negative feeling like that you must rapidly transform that emotion into something that is useful and that mobilises you, such as determination, tenacity, inner strength, or even calm.

Unconscious Identity and Life Vision

Daily immersion in these exercises will keep your levels of energy and passion high, and maintain a focused sense of purpose and direction, giving you the impetus to blast through any obstacles and setbacks that come along.

Repatterning

If you found yourself drifting off course in the past when unexpected events occurred, then repatterning is an excellent technique for installing different habitual responses in these types of situations and will keep you on track and committed.

Overcoming Obstacles and Setbacks

Assuming that you are already using these technologies to transform your mindset and up your game, when we are faced with any obstacle or setback, there are three key things we need to do in that moment:

1. Change the meaning
2. Learn the important lessons
3. Plan

1. Change The Meaning

When things go wrong, many people habitually assume that means failure, and they attach meanings such as "this means I'll never get there", "this proves I can't do it", "this proves I'll always be overweight", and so on.

So first we must change the meaning. Does this mean that you are doomed to a particular fate and that you'll never get what you truly want, or is this actually a really important and useful thing for you?

One of the first important meanings to attach to this event is to recognise that this is part of the journey. You cannot get away with pursuing a big, significant goal, and expect it to be all plain sailing. Unfortunately, a lot of people go off track because that is precisely what they expect. They don't expect to have to grow, develop, or change themselves, their mindset, their approach, and to constantly evolve as they go through this process.

Any goal is a journey of personal development. Goals are people-growing machines. When you achieve a goal you are not the same person as when you started; you *must* grow and develop *in order to get there.*

When you meet an obstacle, manage your internal reactions and say to yourself, "That's OK, I knew I would have to prove my desire and commitment at some point, and this is just one of those times. This is an opportunity for me to prove my worth, it's an opportunity for me to prove how much I want this goal, it's an opportunity for me to grow, to learn, and to get stronger".

Now it is only natural when you are in the thick of a problem to think "Screw the opportunity! I just want this problem to go away, I just want out, fix it!" That's normal, and most people feel that way to begin with. However, the faster you can switch from that thinking to looking for the opportunities and where you need to step up and grow, the easier your life will become, and the more empowered and more at peace you will feel.

People don't get stronger by having an easy life, they get stronger by overcoming adversity. Once you overcome this particular obstacle, you are better off: you're stronger, you have greater ability, more inner resources, and it sets you up to be able to grow to the next stage in life.

So in addition to your own meanings that you can attribute to this event, you can add the following:

> » It is part of the journey, and an essential part of your ultimate success
> » It is an opportunity to learn
> » It is an opportunity to get stronger

2. Learn the Important Lessons

Every obstacle or setback has a learning opportunity, and often a learning *necessity*. Let's use injuries as an example. If you exercise hard enough for long enough, you are almost certainly going to get some kind of niggle, or injury. Perhaps you had errors in your technique you didn't even know about. You go and see a physical therapist, high quality personal trainer, or corrective exercise specialist, and discover that your injury is a result of poor technique, restrictions, poor mobility, poor stability, or movement dysfunction. Exercise technique is not something that you learn once and never have to revisit, it is something that you will continue to improve upon for years to make it both safer, and more effective.

So in this example, learning those important lessons is not only necessary to prevent you making the same mistakes, but it means that you will get better and better results, because with better technique, the exercise becomes more effective.

In many instances, you will not discover the important lessons on your own. You will often need to hire help, or educate yourself in some way. My preference is to hire help. You don't know what you don't know, and hiring an expert can save you years of struggle.

Problem Thinking vs Outcome Thinking

At this point it is important to understand the difference between learning, and what we call problem thinking.

Problem thinking is where you focus on the problem, the costs incurred, how bad things are going to be as a result, and who is to blame.

Outcome thinking focuses on the outcomes you want to achieve, and how you are going to get from where you are now to where you want to be. It is focused on the future, and moving forwards in a positive direction.

Recognise that this is very similar to Towards and Away From thinking. As we discussed, any time you feel stuck or have a problem, it is very easy to start talking in Away From language. If you ask yourself "what do I want?" and you immediately think "I just wish this hadn't happened" and spend all your time and energy focusing on how terrible things are now, who is to blame, and so on, then you are stuck in problem thinking, and need to rapidly switch to outcome thinking.

Once again, it is only natural to have a moment of anger, an outburst, or to be briefly upset. But the moment you notice that you are in a negative state, focusing on the problem and thinking in Away Froms, you must train yourself to change your state rapidly into a positive and empowering one that supports your goals, the person you want to be, and the life you want to live. Focus on outcomes and use Towards language. This skill is a muscle that you need to exercise. The more you use it the more you develop your own inner strength, the more success you will have, the more you will feel in control of yourself and your life, and the happier you will feel.

There is a big difference between objectively reviewing what happened in order to learn something useful and make new distinctions so that you can get better in the future, and problem thinking, where you just feel bad but get no benefit.

Learning From Mistakes

Remember our discussion on mental rehearsal. As part of learning from the past, we have to review it. However, if we are talking about things that, upon reflection, were mistakes, or certainly behaviours or responses that we do not want to repeat in the future, then it is critical that we do not represent those memories to ourselves in the same way they originally happened ever again.

Otherwise we are simply using mental rehearsal to reinforce that same behaviour in the future.

This applies to times you may have allowed your mindset to get out of hand, perhaps worrying, feeling overwhelmed, or managing your time poorly, which then led to some form of self-sabotage, such as binge eating, skipping workouts, or using alcohol to manage your state.

Instead, follow these steps:

» Disassociate and play the situation from a third person's perspective

» Identify the key things you needed to spot, and the changes in your thoughts, focus, meanings, and actions that would ensure you create a favourable outcome in similar situations in the future

» Replay a new experience of that event, this time associated, with yourself thinking, feeling and responding in exactly the way you want, ultimately leading to a favourable outcome. Replay this several times, making it more and more vivid to fully embed and install this new response

3. Plan

As part of your outcome thinking, you may need to come up with a new plan, update your old one, or introduce some intermediary goals or targets.

Using the injury example, you can no longer follow your original training plan and path of progression for the time being. Instead you go off on a bit of a tangent for a while to do the corrective exercise and therapy. Then once you are back on track and continuing with your journey, the chances are that you will be that much more successful thanks to that slight detour.

Motivation

In order to do all this work – facing obstacles and setbacks as they occur, managing your mindset, learning, and planning – it's important you actually want the outcome in the first place. So this brings us all the way back to our motivation chapter when we were talking about what keeps somebody on track. Your goal needs to be an integral part of your identity, who you are, and the life you are committed to living. Once again it's really important that you've already done the work earlier in this book: you are clear on your Push and Pull motivation, and have set goals that genuinely and thoroughly excite you to your very core, that are a true reflection of your core identity, and that you'll do whatever it takes to achieve.

Foreseeable Obstacles and Setbacks

Many of the challenges you will face are predictable. If you know that there are certain hazards that are likely to occur, then plan your responses to them in advance, so that rather than being reactive and on the back foot, you can be proactive.

Here are some of the key obstacles on a body transformation programme that most people are likely to face. For each one, decide how you will respond in terms of your mental response and your physical response. What mental state will you choose that would be most useful, how will you choose to respond emotionally, and what meanings can you associate to that event? As far as your physical response is concerned what are the actions, behaviours and steps you will take to navigate your way around this issue?

Injuries

If you get injured, how will you respond emotionally? What meanings will you attach to it? How will you go about resolving it? How will you invest time and/or money in getting better? What decisions are you going to make?

For example, in the past, many people may have gone completely off plan with their diet whenever they have been injured, taking the attitude of "well I'm not training anyway, so I might as well eat whatever the hell I want". Is that the mindset you want?

Equally they may use it as an excuse not to train at all, this time taking the attitude of "well I'm injured now, I can't do anything". There are very few injuries where you can't do anything at all. Most of them can be worked around. You might need the help of a professional to guide you with that, but there is almost always something you can do.

Mistakes

How will you respond when you make mistakes? As far as meanings are concerned, it is important to recognise the importance, and the place mistakes have in your success.

Success comes from making good decisions.

Good decisions come from good judgement.

Good judgement comes from experience.

Experience comes from bad judgement.

You have to make mistakes. Many of the most successful people in the world are those who have made the most mistakes.

What does making a mistake mean to you? Failure, evidence of your limitations, proof that you can't do it, or that you aren't good enough? Or is it part of the journey, part of learning, an essential part of success? Does it mean you are now one step closer to success? Stronger, with better experience?

If you slip up on your diet in a challenging environment, and you eat something that perhaps you shouldn't have, does that mean you are a failure and you'll never succeed? Or does it mean that there is something you need to learn? Is this actually a great opportunity to install more successful behaviours in a way that not only makes you more successful in this particular environment, but in a way that also spills over and produces benefits in other areas of your life? Do you actually need to go back to your motivation, revisit your goal-setting, or your life vision, and make that much clearer in your mind so that you can make better choices and decision in the future?

You *are* going to make mistakes. The question is how will you respond? Decide ahead of time how you will handle mistakes mentally, emotionally, and behaviourally.

Travelling

Many people use travelling a lot on business, or a long commute as an excuse for going off track. You'll often hear people saying things like, "Well there's just nothing available that's good to eat!" Instead, plan for it in advance. Can you take food with you? Can you research where you are going to find the foods that will keep you on track? Can you make the best of a bad situation, and rather than going completely off the rails, make reasonable, appropriate choices based on the options available?

Peer Pressure

This is an extremely common obstacle for many people starting out in a body transformation programme. It can come from anyone in your life - colleagues, family, even friends. When you make a big change to your behaviour and your lifestyle, it can be a shock to some people because you are behaving out of character as far as they are concerned. Also, when you set a new goal, step up, face your fears, and take action, you can end up inadvertently highlighting other people's weaknesses, faults, shortcomings, their inability to plan, and their lack of desire. They sit around and want, and you have seriously annoyed them by doing. Action frequently offends the inactive.

We would hope that people would use your example as an inspiration to improve their own lives, but unfortunately it's a lot easier to tear you down than it is to build themselves up, and sadly that's the choice some people will make.

Sometimes they will be subtle and offer you food as gifts or treats, or perhaps they will express concern for your health, suggesting they are worried about you becoming neurotic or how much time you are spending at the gym.

Other times they will try to use guilt and suggest you are having a negative impact on their lives, and that you're just being selfish.

Or perhaps they may try to bribe, mock, or carefully plant the seeds of doubt or negativity.

How will you respond if this happens to you? Will you get defensive, angry, aggressive, or feel pressured to justify yourself? Or are you going to recognise that is all their stuff, their issues, their problems, and their projections, and remain unaffected? Are you going to change who you hang out with? Are you going to have a frank conversation with some people?

Once again decide ahead of time how you will respond emotionally as well as physically/verbally, depending on the types of peer pressure, comments or influence you may receive.

Others?

What other obstacles or setbacks are you likely to face on your journey? Spend a few moments thinking about some of the possible scenarios that could get in your way, and then repeat this process, deciding how you will respond both internally and externally.

Summary

Obstacles and setbacks are going to happen. They are part of the journey towards any worthwhile goal.

Your ability to manage your state and your emotions will be tested. Be vigilant with applying your state management skills *when* things don't go to plan.

Keep your sights on the big picture. Remember your Life Vision and Unconscious Identity, and *why* your goals are important to you. Obstacles are a test of your commitment to those goals.

Use repatterning to install the way you want to habitually respond to such challenges.

In order to overcome obstacles and setbacks you must:

Change the meaning. Empowering meanings can be found in any situation when you sincerely look for them. These challenges are part of the journey, an opportunity to learn, and an opportunity to get stronger.

Learn the important lessons. Failure to learn the lessons makes it more likely you'll experience the same struggles in the future.

Switch from problem thinking to outcome thinking as quickly as possible.

Remember there is no such thing as failure, there is only feedback and information.

Learn from mistakes. Acknowledge the difference between reliving failure, and learning from mistakes so that you grow and improve.

Plan how you are going to get from where you are now to your goals. Do you need to update your old plan, or create a new one?

Your motivation to put in the work necessary to overcome obstacles and setbacks depends on your desire to achieve your goals in the first place. Remember your goals must be truly exciting and empowering.

Prepare for foreseeable obstacles and setbacks in advance. Prepare what you would *do*, and how you will choose to react *emotionally*.

Chapter 12

Internal Conflicts

What You Will Learn

» Why people engage in seemingly irrational behaviours, and at the same time wish they didn't.

» How internal conflicts are created and where they come from.

» The hidden benefits of irrational behaviours.

» How to resolve internal conflicts forever.

Parts

Any time that someone is engaged in a behaviour, and at the same time wishes they weren't, we can call this an internal conflict. Connirae Andreas, a psychotherapist known for her work in the field of neurolinguistic programming (NLP) developed a beautiful method for working with internal conflicts called core transformations. We can also refer to internal conflicts as "Parts" as people often describe them in that manner:

"Part of me wants this and part of me wants that."

"It's as though part of me takes over."

"There's a part of me I can't control."

Internal conflicts and parts are particularly common in dieting and with disordered eating:

"I can't stop binge eating."

"I know I shouldn't eat it but I just can't stop myself."

"Why can't I stick to my diet?"

"I know I need to exercise more, and part of me really wants to, but for some reason I keep sabotaging myself."

How Are Parts Created?

Parts are usually created at a fairly early age, when we encounter a new situation or environment that is confusing or challenging. We don't fully understand how to interpret events or how to respond which leaves us feeling paralysed. In order to bridge this gap in our understanding we create a belief which indicates a particular course of action. This at least enables us to respond in some way, which is better than being paralysed by not knowing.

A typical example of a parts issue in body transformations is the person who wants to get fitter, leaner and healthier, but at the same time can't stop eating chocolate. There are all sorts of different ways they could develop this internal conflict but here is just one example:

They grow up in a turbulent household and don't have the most stable, or nurturing environment. This might be as seemingly insignificant as fighting with siblings and the parents not getting involved, or as destructive as an alcoholic or abusive parent. What matters is the internal world of the child - how they feel, how they interpret things, and the options they perceive as being available.

They desperately want to reduce a negative emotion (fear, anxiety etc) or access a positive emotion (e.g. love, connection, security) in the best way they have available. They experiment with food and discover that it temporarily distracts them from the stress, and provides them with some degree of comfort.

This may not give them the perfect outcome, but some state change is better than no change. This is a reasonable response because at that stage in their life, and at that age, it is the best, and quite possibly the only option they have for meeting their emotional needs, based on their understanding of themselves, their capabilities, other people, what's possible, and their limited model of the world.

They may have learnt to use chocolate from someone else or simply through experimentation, but they would have tried this behaviour in a number of situations until they discovered that it produced consistent results. Then through repetition their brain strengthens that neural pathway, and stores eating as the most rapid, reliable, and effective way of changing their state when things feel too stressful and out of control.

This behaviour gets validated and stored unconsciously as the correct response in these types of situations, and the beliefs created around it become stored as the truth. We mistake these assumptions, approximations, and best guesses as reality instead of a useful set of approximations that got us out of a difficult situation back when we were a lot younger and didn't know any better.

The brain makes these types of neurological short cuts whenever it is learning and encountering new situations. Generalisations are a valuable time-saving process that enable us to survive and react automatically instead of having to stop and assess what's happening each time. However, after a while some of them may become outdated, and can end up causing more problems than they solve.

In the case of our chocolate eater, as an adult this person uses overeating to comfort and connect with themselves. They think of chocolate as a reward for a day completed. Perhaps during the day this person has a very busy life that is focused on others. Maybe they work long hours in a hospital, and on top of this they have small children to take care of. They love their children and their job, but by the end of the day they need to feel comforted, rewarded, and to reconnect with themselves after giving so much to others during the day. This triggers the part of them responsible for resolving this problem - the chocolate eating part.

What this part really wants for them is a sense of comfort and security, and a way to feel connected and loved. Eating chocolate was merely a method for attempting to achieve this outcome based on the beliefs and under-standing of a small child. As this person gets older they gain new experiences and learn more about themselves, other people, and the world. However, because that part is now fully automated and operating independently it continues to function with the same set of beliefs and understanding that were present at the age when it was created.

Unfortunately, this person is now very overweight and desperately wants to lose weight, get lean, fit and healthy, and feel better about themselves. But every time they try to improve their diet they sabotage themselves with chocolate over and over again.

Positive Intention

As part of resolving this process it is vital to understand and appreciate that all behaviour, no matter how illogical or destructive it may seem, has a positive intention at its core. It is designed to give you an important benefit at an unconscious level. The origin of this positive intention is usually in one of the following categories:

» To **protect** you from something

» To **prevent** something from happening

» To **provide** you with something

This is a fundamental benefit and need that you have at a deeper level. The only issue is that the part you created to provide you with that benefit is hampered by the beliefs and understanding that were present at the age at which you created it. As a result, the choices and behaviours that result are no longer in alignment with the present. In the example above, the part this person created doesn't want them to eat chocolate as a core intention, it wants to give them love and connection.

By identifying the positive intention of the part, we can update this person's model of the world and help them develop new behaviours that meet their needs in ways that are more effective and congruent.

Connecting and Communicating with The Part

Since the behaviour we are seeking to resolve was developed to a point where it was fully automated and fully unconscious, it continued to operate independently. One of the things that will amplify this isolation even further is hating the part. This is a common response since we don't understand it, why it was created, and what its positive intentions were. We don't like the consequences, and it feels out of our control.

In order to resolve this internal conflict, we need to connect with that part of us, understand it, and integrate it with the rest of us so that it can have access to updated information, our new model of the world, and new possibilities.

Unfortunately, if you hate that part and mistreat it, the dynamics of this relationship only serves to isolate that part even further and prevent the integration you need.

Before we can learn the part's core intentions and fully integrate it with the rest of us, we *must* establish better communication with it. It is vital to genuinely and authentically acknowledge and thank that part, and even to apologise to it, before we can hope to understand it. This step must be genuine and sincere so that that part can learn to trust us again. Only then can we communicate with it effectively and discover its positive intentions.

Imagine if you were negotiating between two countries at war. You tell one "we love you guys, we think you're great and agree with everything you do". You then approach the second and say "we hate you lot, you're disgusting and everything you do is wrong". What are the changes of resolving that conflict? Zero! You *must* treat both parties with equal importance, value, and love.

Exercise: Internal Conflict Resolution

Step 1: Relaxation

Get yourself somewhere quiet and private where you can remain undisturbed for approximately half an hour. Sit in a comfortable position, close your eyes, and spend a few minutes relaxing and going internal. Focus on your breathing and allow it to become deeper and slower. Passively pay attention to what you can hear and what you can feel in your body as you relax deeper.

Step 2: Connect with the part

Get in touch with and connect with the part you want to reintegrate. Notice in which area of your body this behaviour resides. How is it represented? What does it look like, feel like, or sound like? Trust your unconscious reaction. Just notice what spontaneously comes to mind.

Step 3: Acknowledge and thank the part

Remind yourself of how and why we get parts. Remind yourself that this is a part that was created in response to a difficult situation. At that time, it was the best and probably the only sensible and appropriate response. Ever since then it has simply been carrying out a set of instructions it was given a long time ago.

Notice the admirable qualities you can already recognise in this part. It is reliable and dependable. It has extraordinary resilience and tenacity. Imagine what it will be like when you are able to direct those qualities towards what you really want in life. That's what this part can do for you.

All this part has ever wanted was to provide you with something valuable and important - something you need. Even though it's been rejected, hated and repulsed, it's so committed to getting something really valuable in your life that it has not given up on you. How many times would you need to be told to "**** off!" before you gave up on someone? Yet this part has worked tirelessly and thanklessly to help you, in spite of how you've treated it.

Even though you may not fully understand this part yet, genuinely and authentically thank it. Do this out loud now. Notice how this feels. Make sure it feels congruent and meaningful before moving on.

If you have mistreated this part and been nasty or hateful towards it in the past, then also apologise to it.

As you acknowledge and thank this part, notice how it changes the way that you see that part and the way that you feel towards it. You may notice changes in where it is located, and what it looks, feels, or sounds like.

Step 4: Positive Intention

Ask that part "What is your positive intention? What is it that you have been trying to provide for me that is positive through doing this behaviour?"

Trust your unconscious processes and notice the answer that automatically and spontaneously pops into your mind. Acknowledge and thank the part for answering, and write down the answer.

For example, you may get answers such as "to feel in control", "protection from being hurt", "to feel safe", "to feel love" and so on. This is the first level, the first layer of understanding.

You will now repeat a three-part process to discover deeper and deeper layers of understanding:

Imagine yourself experiencing that positive intention totally and completely, in every area of your life, whenever you want and need it.

Ask that part, "If I were totally and completely in control (replace in control with whichever positive intention has been identified), then what does that provide me with that is even more important?". You may get an answer such as confidence, freedom, energy or something else. This is the next level of understanding. Write the answer down.

Acknowledge and thank the part for wanting to give you this positive intention. Then return to the first step and imagine yourself experiencing this new positive intention totally and completely.

Continue this process until it feels like you reach the highest, most profound level. For example, you could go through the following levels:

» To feel in control

» Confidence

» The ability to love unconditionally

» To help others love unconditionally

» To find peace

» To achieve enlightenment

» To help others find enlightenment

As you ask these questions and go through each level, go with your gut, your first response, without filtering. Take your time with each step to do it thoroughly, to feel it completely, and to allow time for your unconscious to process and respond to each level.

Once again, notice how the way in which you represent that part is transformed unconsciously with each layer of understanding. Notice how it changes location, appearance, feel, or sound.

When you get to your highest positive intention, let that part know that you fully agree with its positive purpose. Thank it again, and notice how it feels to finally recognise what it really has wanted for you all this time. From now on refer to it as its highest-level intention.

Step 5: Start from the highest intention and work backwards

Imagine yourself experiencing your highest intention totally and completely. Then bring that feeling back into the positive intention preceding it. Using the above example, feel yourself helping others to achieve enlightenment, and then bring that feeling back into achieving enlightenment for yourself. Notice what has changed now. What can you appreciate? What are you aware of? What do you now know to be true?

With this new level of understanding and new experience, bring this feeling back into the positive intention preceding that one. Using the above example again, bring the combined experience of achieving enlightenment for yourself and for others back into the experience of finding peace. Repeat this process, taking your time to feel each experience in turn. Feel how it is has changed, how it integrates within you, and what you now understand, before bringing all this back into the next positive intention before it and so on.

Once you get back to the start notice the integration you feel. Many people have intriguing sensations at this point. Simply notice what happens and allow it to happen. Also, notice the new insights and perspective you have now and how differently things feel.

Step 6: Future pace

Imagine your future with this new integration in place. How does having that right now transform your experience of the world? Imagine yourself in vivid detail going through the coming weeks, months, and years, fully integrated and able to act from the best in you. Look forward with eager anticipation, knowing that everything is about to change for the better.

When you take the time to do this exercise properly, thoroughly, and open yourself to your unconscious responses the results are profound. This is an approach you can take with any recurring problem or emotional blockage. The possibilities are limitless. The key is to relax, have fun with it and be spontaneous. Trust that your unconscious mind knows best, and knows more about you than you do. Once all your unconscious processes are integrated and aligned with each other everything becomes so much easier, and all your behaviours and choices become congruent with each other.

If you have had a part of you that has sabotaged your fat loss or body transformation attempts, that you wish you could change but feel powerless to do so, and that feels out of your control, then use this technique. Reconnect with that part, discover the intentions that lie beneath the behaviour, and then fully integrate that part so that you can find new ways of achieving that ultimate positive intention without the negative consequences of the old destructive behaviour.

Ultimately your brain doesn't want you to binge eat, or sabotage your fitness goals. It is trying to provide you with a higher-level intention. That old behaviour is simply an outdated vehicle for attempting to meet those needs. By discovering the higher-level intention, you can help your mind to come up with alternative ways of meeting those needs more effectively, without the old sabotage behaviours. When you properly connect with that part, acknowledge and thank it, understand it and its positive intentions, and then integrate it with the rest of your unconscious, these changes happen easily and naturally.

Summary

Parts are created in response to a confusing or challenging environment.

They are reasonable because at that age, based on our experience, our understanding of ourselves, other people, our own capabilities, what's possible, and our limited model of the world, they are the best, and quite possibly the only choice available.

Over time the behaviour generated by the part can become paradoxical to its original intention and it can end up causing more harm than good.

All parts, and all irrational or seemingly illogical behaviours have a positive intention at their core. They are trying to provide us with a benefit at an unconscious level. This is usually to protect, prevent or provide.

It is important to distinguish the part and its positive intention from the behaviour.

Before we can fully understand the part's positive intention, and resolve the internal conflict, we *must* genuinely and authentically acknowledge and thank that part first.

Once we acknowledge and thank the part, and understand its positive intentions, we can fully integrate that part with the rest of us in a way that enables us to retain all the core benefits, with none of the negative consequences of the old limiting behaviours.

Follow the internal conflict resolution exercise to resolve internal conflicts.

Chapter 13 Get a Coach

If you have struggled to make the significant changes to your body and your life that you are after, or if you want to really take your results to the next level, hire a coach.

Very often people are hesitant to invest the time, money, and energy required for high level coaching. They have fears and doubts such as "Will it really work? Is it worth it? Surely I can figure it out on my own?" and so on. These concerns are all valid, and legitimate questions to ask.

In my opinion, the fastest way to get ahead in life, and to build the body, the life, the happiness and the fulfilment you want is through coaching. The most forward thinking, fastest growing, and innovative companies invest 10-15% of their income on professional development every year. If you treat yourself in the same way, you too can have the same rate of success and development.

Many people will hire a coach, therapist, or trainer to help them resolve one particular issue. Examples include when someone wants to resolve an eating disorder, improve their self-esteem, get through their marital problems, overcome depression, or get better at public speaking. However, coaching is not only how you get rid of the obstacles and problems you are stuck with, it is how you develop and get more and more out of yourself and your life. You can take yourself to levels of success, excitement, energy, and passion that you never thought possible with consistent coaching. Why settle for an adequate life when you can have an extraordinary one?

For this reason, I invest in coaching and mentoring every year. The leading professionals in my network do the same. My coaches have coaches of their own. You will notice that the most successful people in society all have coaches.

The best athletes, singers, and sports professionals in the world will all have coaches. In these examples, the coach won't even be as good at running, singing, or playing that sport as the athlete they are coaching. But the coach will provide them with things they can't get by themselves: an external, unbiased perspective of their performance, and experience and knowledge from fields they are not trained in, such as peak performance and psychology.

People who stagnate in life, who go through the motions without resolving their problems, or without growing or improving, tend to try and fix everything on their own.

Sometimes they try to figure it out on their own using their existing mindset. But of course, this approach is limited by their own model of the world, their beliefs, perspective, experience, and unconscious strategies. Remember the spelling strategy? There are so many other systems of operation that occur at the uncon-scious level. You don't know what you don't know.

People also try to educate themselves on their own issues. This can work, but it requires relentless persistence, commitment and hard work to do so. Once again you don't know what you don't know, so you may have to read 100 books to find the one that identifies the specific approach you need to resolve your particular issue. Then you need the self-awareness to notice that specific issue in yourself, and then you need to do the work. Unfortu-nately, most people who take this approach end up with highly-educated bookshelves, but actually read about 5% of the content, and continue for years without resolving their own personal issues.

Even for those who do commit to doing this work, are you going to do this for every single issue in your life? The expert you hire has invested years studying, thousands of hours working with clients, learning, making mistakes, refining their approach and honing their skill so that they can help resolve your issue as quickly as possible.

The one thing you can never get back is time. Investing in experts can save you years of struggle. By investing in experts consistently, you can surge through life growing faster than you ever thought possible.

Some of the other benefits of hiring a coach include:

» They can point out your **blind spots**. We all have patterns of thought and behaviour that occur at the unconscious level. Once again, you don't know what you don't know. An effective coach will point these out and help you to change them where necessary

» **Interventions, and breakthroughs** - a quality coach will help you resolve long standing issues that have sabotaged your progress or inhibited your success and happiness. These could include habits, persistent thoughts, feelings or behaviours that feel out of your control, addictions, fear, procrastination, and other struggles

» **Strategies** - a coach will teach you the strategies you need to get the results you have hired them for. These could be internal strategies for managing your own thoughts and feelings or organising your internal world, or external strategies for improving your effectiveness and productivity in a particular environment

» **Accountability** - a coach will keep you on track and accountable, making sure you live up to the commitment you made at the start.

» **Support** - a coach will provide you with the support you need to remain on track, consistent, and to push through any fears or wobbles you might have along the way.

Occasionally you might invest in a course or a coach who doesn't deliver what you hoped or what you expected. If you source your coach wisely this is unlikely, but it can happen. If it does, put it down as part of the cost of personal growth. If you are prepared to continue to invest a percentage of your income every year in personal growth, it will be a drop in the ocean, and the benefits, health, wealth, happiness, fulfilment, and growth you will experience in your life will be exponentially more than the money you have invested.

When it comes down to it, the main concerns people have about the financial investment or questions about "will it work? is it worth it?" and so on are ultimately a reflection of their own fears and doubts. When you source your coaches wisely, you will see from their track record that they can deliver the results you are looking for. Those results are dependent on three things:

» The quality of their content

» The quality of their coaching

» The client's application, and commitment to follow through

Their results and track record are testimony that their quality of content and coaching is high enough. The one thing any coach cannot guarantee is the client's application. You have to do the work! If you approach any course, programme, or coaching that you invest in with the attitude of "I will make this work! No ifs, ands or buts, I will do whatever it takes. Whatever happens, I will find a way!" then how can you not succeed?

The trouble is people have too many reference experiences of not following through on their commitments. Or they buy into the learned helplessness beliefs we mentioned earlier about the permanence of a problem.

Ultimately, if you have an area of your life you want to improve, and if it is truly important to you, get a coach. When you hire that coach, make the decision to do whatever it takes to get the result you want. The Latin word decision literally means to cut off from. Cut off from any possibility other than success. Burn your bridges and give yourself no option to go back on your word. When you approach an issue or a goal with that degree of commitment, and a willingness to do whatever it takes to succeed, success becomes inevitable.

Chase Life

Chase Life is a high-end coaching programme designed and delivered by myself and female-fat-loss expert Rachel Guy. It is built as a body transformation programme, but tackles the source of what needs to change for someone to achieve a transformation that lasts and that makes them truly happy.

It is a programme for women, designed to help them make profound, revolutionary changes in themselves and in their lives. We help women discover the real reasons they are not losing weight or why they are struggling with their fat loss attempts and help them break through these plateaus in ways that produce benefits far beyond transforming their body.

We have a range of clients with a variety of goals but most of our clients broadly fit one of the following categories:

» Binge eaters and emotional eaters or those who struggle with control around food

» Perfectionists and over-analysers, often professional, successful women, but who also struggle with stress, frustration, and overwhelm

» Women who struggle with low self-esteem, low self-worth, lack of confidence, or anxiety issues

» Women who, on face value, appear to have it all. They have all the boxes ticked but for some reason remain unhappy and unfulfilled

» Women who genuinely are happy and already have good results in their health, fitness, and happiness, but want to take their life and their results to the next level, to truly chase life

We do this both online via exclusive, application only coaching programmes, as well as premium level retreats and seminar programmes.

This is an advanced and truly transformative programme which requires a high level of commitment and readiness to change. Chase Life is by application only. We need to make sure that everyone who comes through Chase Life meets the following criteria:

» They will be a positive member of the group. It is vital that every member of the group is open, honest, and forthcoming. We are very protective of the supportive environment we have created

» They are coachable, open to feedback and new ways of doing things

» They are completely committed to massive personal change and back this up with action

» They are ready to face confronting challenges

» They are ready to work hard on themselves and their personal growth.

So, if you struggle with...

» Binge eating

» Emotional eating

» Disordered eating

» Perfectionism

- » Stress

- » Overwhelm

- » Anxiety

- » Low self-esteem

- » Poor confidence

or

- » if you lack purpose, feel unhappy, or unfulfilled

- » if you want to take your life and your results from good to amazing

and

- » you are totally committed to transforming yourself and your life, then apply for Chase Life now. Go to www.joinchaselife.com, fill out the application, and we will arrange a consultation with you.

Acknowledgements

First I would like to thank my wife Rachel for being the rock in my life, my best friend and soulmate. Also, not only for being my other half in life, but also in business, and without whom Chase Life would not exist.

Secondly, I would like to thank the geniuses who have been my mentors and coaches over the years: Phil Parker, Stephen Brooks, Richard Bandler, Anthony Robbins, and Cloe Madanes.

Finally, I would like to thank the clients and everyone I have worked with, from whom I have learnt so much, and whose courage to grow continues to inspire me to this day.

The Author

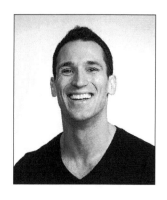

David Godfrey has become one of the UK's most in-demand and influential coaches, with over 15 years of industry experience as a Mindset and Performance Coach.

An NLP master practitioner, hypnotherapist and life coach, David has worked with a wide variety of conditions including depression, chronic fatigue, disordered and compulsive eating, phobias and addiction. He has a reputation as a direct and innovative coach, able to produce rapid and lasting changes with his clients.

David dedicated his early career to body transformations, combining mindset coaching with personal training. With an exceptional skill set he developed unique and powerful systems for helping people create sustainable and life-changing transformations that work, despite the challenges that people often face in their lives and in themselves.

David has since expanded the scope of his practice to help people on a larger scale, specialising in binge eating, emotional eating, stress, overwhelm, anxiety, perfectionism, low self-esteem, and depression.

For contact details and to follow David online go to:
www.joinchaselife.com
www.david-godfrey.com
www.facebook.com/david.godfrey.page
www.youtube.com/user/dxgodfrey
www.instagram.com/dxgodfrey
www.twitter.com/dxgodfrey
www.linkedin.com/in/dxgodfrey

Printed in Great Britain
by Amazon